HOW TO
SUCCESSFULLY WITH

MIGRAINE
THE DRUG FREE WAY

SUE DYSON

Wellhouse Publishing Ltd

First published in 1995 as The Migraine Diet Book by Sheldon Press

This revised and updated edition is published in Great Britain
in 2004 by
Wellhouse Publishing Ltd
31 Middle Bourne Lane
Lower Bourne
Farnham, Surrey GU10 3NH

DISCLAIMER

The aim of this book is to provide general information only and
should not be treated as a substitute for the medical advice of
your doctor or any other health care professional. The publisher
and author is not responsible or liable for any diagnosis made by
a reader based on the contents of this book. Always consult your
doctor if you are in any way concerned about your health.

A catalogue record for this book is available from the British Library

ISBN 1 903784 17 4

Printed and bound in Great Britain by
Creative Print & Design Group, Middlesex UB7 0LW

Contents

Introduction   7

1   What's in a migraine?   9

2   Why watch your diet?   23

3   Finding your food triggers (I)   35

4   Finding your food triggers (II)   47

5   Migraine? No problem!   67

6   A menu for living   81

7   Migraine and slimming   95

8   Migraine and children 101

    Further Reading 113

    Useful Addresses 115

    Index 118

About the author

Sue Dyson is an experienced writer on health, self-help and business subjects; and as a lifelong migraine sufferer the subject of this book is very dear to her heart. In fact, it is true to say that most of what is in it, she has tested on herself.

Sue was born and brought up on Merseyside, and began nurse training which she was forced to give up because of a spinal injury. She subsequently trained as a French translator, and is possibly the only person ever to have become 'Secretary of the Year' without actually working as a secretary!

When not writing non-fiction, Sue translates French novels and is perhaps best known as novelist Zö Barnes. Her light-hearted romances are set in and around Cheltenham, where she lives with her husband Simon and four cats: Grizzle, Jupiter, Domino and Pizza. She also writes a weekly column for the local newspaper and in her spare time is a semi-professional singer.

Introduction

Imagine someone is trying to drill a hole in your head, right through one of your eyes. Imagine your stomach is heaving, your sight disturbed by weird effects of light and shade. Imagine there are pins and needles in your fingers and toes, and your brain is so confused that you can't get out the words you want to say.

Imagine you have migraine.

That is perhaps an extreme description of what it is like to have a migraine attack, but if you are a sufferer it is a fair bet that you will recognise some of the symptoms. Even if you are one of the 'lucky' ones who only suffer from sickness and a throbbing, one-sided headache, that can be enough to incapacitate you for days on end.

Perhaps worst of all is the lack of understanding, not to mention the abuse of the word 'migraine' as a cover-all for anyone who fancies an illicit day off sick. Slight headache? 'I've got a migraine.' Hangover? 'Sorry boss, I won't be in today – I've got one of my migraines again'. Before you know it, half the world is suffering in silence and the other half thinks the first half is putting it on.

This book is written by someone who does understand. I can say that with my hand on my heart, because I have suffered with migraine ever since I was a child. I'm not sure when I had my first attack, but I do clearly recall being very poorly on my seventh birthday and wondering why chocolate didn't make me feel any better!

These days there are many excellent and effective medical treatments for migraine – both for treating the symptoms and for preventing the attacks in the first place. However, these don't all work for everybody all the time, and they are not the main focus of this book.

Migraine – The Drug-Free Way aims to point to a different route for anyone who feels that conventional medicine isn't the whole of the answer. It can, of course, be used in conjunction with conventional medical treatment, and indeed I would advise anyone to consult his or her GP before embarking on any kind of self-help approach.

This book looks in particular at the dietary component that bedevils many migraine sufferers' lives. It's not just a question of cheese, red wine and chocolate – there can be a much more complex pattern of food intolerances and sensitivities at work, and if these can be identified real improvement can be achieved without large doses of prescription drugs.

Even if it turns out that you aren't one of the sufferers for whom diet is an important factor, following the guidelines for healthy eating, exercise and relaxation can only help to improve your general health, wellbeing and morale. And it's surprising how much better we all feel when our bodies are well maintained and our attitudes upbeat.

I can't promise any miracle cures or overnight successes; but as a fellow-sufferer whose own symptoms have markedly improved through an holistic approach, I can certainly assure you that it's worth a try.

Here's wishing you the best of health.

Sue Dyson

Chapter One

What's in a migraine?

If you have just been diagnosed as having migraine, you may well be feeling frightened. On the other hand, you may even be feeling slightly relieved. At last that periodic agony you've been suffering has been given a name, and at least you know it isn't going to kill you, however bad you may feel at the height of an attack. You are now ready to work your way through this book, which will show you ways to identify and eliminate any dietary element in your attacks.

If you are suffering from bad or frequent headaches but have not yet found out why, please make an appointment to see your doctor immediately. Most headaches are readily treatable, and just talking to someone about them can ease the tension that tends to make them so much more unbearable. In any case, it simply isn't worth taking chances with your health. Self-help is designed to complement conventional medicine, not to replace it. Once you know what is causing your pain, you can begin to learn how to cope with it – and in time, to overcome it.

In this chapter we're going to take a look at what migraine is and isn't. There are many types of headache, and each responds to different forms of treatment – although dietary therapy can be helpful in a wide range of cases, not just migraine.

What is migraine?

Relatively little is known for certain about migraine, although scientists have been carrying out research into it for over a century. However, a number of facts have been observed and theories developed.

The 'vascular' theory
Scientists describe migraine as a 'vascular headache' – in other words, a migraine attack involves changes in the behaviour of the

blood vessels. In the stage leading up to an attack, the blood vessels around the brain become constricted (narrowed), and subsequently dilate (expand) to many times their normal size. This phase of dilation is when the pain is felt and you get that familiar throbbing, pounding migraine headache.

The pain is usually one-sided, and sufferers often say that it seems to be throbbing in time with the pulse. Each beat of the heart pumps more blood into the already congested blood vessels of the head, causing more pain. It used to be thought that it was this unusual activity in the blood vessels which actually caused a migraine attack, but nowadays most doctors believe that this is just a symptom resulting from much more complex changes in the brain itself.

The 'neurological' theory

Most specialists now favour this theory, which states that migraine involves chemical changes in the brain. These affect the activity of nerves, which carry messages about sensations like pain. A sort of wave of inactivity called a 'nerve storm', may pass over the surface of the brain just before an attack.

One of the chemicals thought to be involved is serotonin, the levels of which seem to fall during an attack. Serotonin is associated with constriction of the blood vessels and acts on the brainstem, the part of the brain at the top of the spine, which stops us feeling pain. Doctors talk about a 'pain gate', which is normally kept 'closed' by the brain stem, so we don't suffer pain.

When chemical changes leave the pain gate open, we are likely to suffer migraine attacks. Certain 'triggers', like anxiety, seem to open the pain gate, whereas relaxation techniques can be used to help close it. Other trigger factors, such as eating foods you are sensitive to, or hormonal changes just before a period, combine to make an attack more likely. It is believed that for an attack to take place, there must be a combination of several trigger factors; for example, stress + hormonal changes + trigger food = migraine.

On the plus side, it's important to recognize that pain is an important warning sign. Many experts believe that an attack may be your body's way of making you stop and switch off when you have been overdoing things: a bit like blowing an electrical fuse.

Types of migraine

Migraine has been divided up into different types, or classifications.

Migraine without aura
This used to be called 'common migraine', and it is the commonest form of the illness. However, it is much more than just a headache. The National Headache Foundation in America classifies it as:
Severe, one-sided throbbing pain, often accompanied by nausea, vomiting, cold hands, tremor, dizziness, sensitivity to sound and light.

The severe, one-sided headache may come on without warning, and may come on at regular intervals – e.g. once a week or once a month. It can also occur in response to certain circumstances or stimuli – for example, environmental factors, stress, or eating certain foods.

What happens in a migraine attack?
During an attack, most sufferers find that all they want to do is lie or sit quietly in the dark, and try to sleep. A few say that when the attack is not too severe they prefer to move about and keep going, as this helps to make the attack go away more quickly.

They find that if they give in to the pain, it seems to cause them more distress.

Symptoms may include:

- throbbing one-sided headache
- nausea and/or vomiting
- sensitivity to light
- diarrhoea
- frequent urination or fluid retention
- feeling very hot or very cold
- heightened sensitivity to sounds and smells
- speech problems
- general malaise.

Migraine with aura
This used to be called 'classical migraine'. Like common migraine, this involves a powerful, one-sided headache with nausea and/or vomiting, dislike of strong light, loud noises and pungent smells.

The difference between this form of migraine and common migraine lies in the 'aura', a set of internal warning signs, which tell the sufferer that an attack is on the way. These signs vary widely from individual to individual, but they generally last between a few minutes and an hour, and stop when the headache starts. They take place in the pre-headache (prodromal) stage when the blood vessels in the head are constricted.

Early treatment is important, and you may be able to abort an attack if you recognize the warning signs and act quickly enough.

Aura symptoms may include:
visual disturbances e.g. flashing lights, spots, zig-zags, coloured stars, blind spots, double vision, temporary loss of vision

- pins and needles, weakness or numbness in hands or feet (especially on one side), temporary paralysis (very rare)
- blurred vision
- changes in the perception of objects, the world, other people, even yourself (known as the 'Alice in Wonderland syndrome')
- slurred speech, or difficulty in expressing your thoughts
- heightened sense of smell
- nasty taste in the mouth

These symptoms may be alarming, but it's important to realize that they are not dangerous. They may also be useful to you, as a sufferer, as they give you advance warning of an attack and may help you to abort it or reduce its severity by prompt treatment. Many sufferers find that certain types of food and drink are helpful in this early stage of an attack, and we will be looking at this in a later section of the book.

Some people may also have earlier warning signs, which manifest themselves the previous day. You may find that your family and friends notice them before you do, so it's worth asking them to jot down any changes in your behaviour and moods. This may help to pinpoint times when you're likely to have an attack, and perhaps to identify any foods which may be making you ill (symptoms of which may take up to 36 hours to appear).

These earlier signs may include:

- strange sensations
- hunger, thirst, food cravings
- mood changes (anxiety, elation, subtle mood-swings)
- feeling full of energy and wellbeing
- lassitude
- premonitions
- yawning

These very early signs may also precede an attack of common migraine.

Aura without headache

This used to be called 'migraine equivalents'.

Curiously enough, not all migraine attacks involve a headache. Sometimes the sufferer has only the aura, and not the headache, which usually follows. Although this may seem preferable, some migraineurs (migraine sufferers) say they find the aura symptoms distressing in themselves.

Cluster headaches

These are often grouped together with migraines, although they aren't really a form of migraine at all.

They are excruciatingly painful, and come in 'clusters' lasting six to twelve weeks. There can be several attacks in a day. Sufferers feel the need to move during an attack, and may pace up and down, hitting their heads against the wall. (Most migraine sufferers prefer to remain very still.) The pain affects one eye only, which goes red and waters. The corresponding nostril also waters but the other side of the face is unaffected and looks normal.

Cluster headache tends to be associated with middle-aged men who have smoked, but there are also many female sufferers. Alcohol may trigger an attack, but only in the cluster period.

Mixed and combination headaches

It is quite possible to switch between common and classical

migraine, and you may also alternate between migraine and muscle tension headaches, sometimes experiencing 'mixed' attacks with features of both conditions. An attack may start off resembling a tension headache and then develop into a full-blown migraine attack. Alternatively, you may have a migraine attack which eases off and then turns into a long-drawn-out tension headache. In some cases, sufferers may find that they are never headache-free.

When a migraine attack continues, with headaches and vomiting, for many days, this is known as status migranosis, it may need to be treated in hospital as it can lead to dehydration.

Often, people do not seek help from GPs or specialists until they start developing mixed headaches. They can cope with the migraine attacks on their own, but when other headaches are added, find that it is too much to bear.

Non-migraine headaches

Of course, not every headache is a migraine attack, and it's important to be able to recognize the differences. In fact, if you suffer from headaches, migraine isn't the most likely cause of them – only around 10 per cent of the population are migraine sufferers, and around 88 per cent of all headaches are classified as 'tension headaches'.

Tension headaches
This term is very misleading, and it would be better to call them 'muscle contraction headaches'. The pain is caused by sustained contraction of the muscles in the face, neck, shoulders and/or jaw, which in turn affects the nerves of the head and causes pain.

Over a period of time, the muscles may become permanently inelastic, and the pain may become chronic, causing great damage to the quality of the sufferer's life.

The pain is often described as 'dull', 'steady', 'like a helmet', and is often on both sides of the head. It may occur daily. These types of headache can be one-sided, and may be confused with migraine attacks.

Acute attacks are usually triggered by stress or anxiety, and respond well to relaxation and over-the-counter (OTC) drugs.

Chronic attacks are harder to treat, and often do not respond to painkillers. Bad posture, repressed emotions and low blood sugar may all contribute to attacks.

Diet and tension headaches

Although dietary factors are not a major cause of tension headaches, a hectic lifestyle can lead to a poor diet and missed meals. This can lead to problems with blood sugar levels, which in turn cause headaches. A good diet, with regular, nutritious meals, may help to restore good health and wellbeing.

Nervous tension tends to lead to the production of high levels of adrenaline and other 'stress chemicals' in the body. These are designed to prepare the body for a 'flight or fight' response to danger – but one of the side effects is to increase muscle tension.

When we are tense or under pressure, we also tend to drink lots of tea, coffee, cola etc. 'to keep us going'. Unfortunately, these contain lots of caffeine, which can also promote higher levels of these 'stress chemicals', so it makes good sense to reduce your intake.

Analgesic headaches

If you suffer from tension headaches regularly, you may not respond very well to painkillers. When you are in pain and nothing much seems to help, the temptation is to take bigger and bigger doses in the hope that a higher dose will have a greater effect.

Obviously, taking large amounts of painkillers can cause serious health problems. Too much aspirin could give you a peptic ulcer, and an overdose (even a relatively small one) of paracetamol could lead to irreversible liver damage and death.

What's more, taking regular doses of painkillers like aspirin and paracetamol can actually cause 'rebound' headaches. The same applies to migraine drugs such as ergotamine, which can cause migraine-like symptoms if too much is taken. This is also a problem with many proprietary pain-relievers that contain caffeine in addition to aspirin, ibuprofen and/or paracetamol.

Where possible, avoid taking drugs as preventive treatments, and try to prevent your headaches by means of a more relaxed lifestyle, gentle exercise and better nutrition. We shall be looking at the elements of a healthy diet in Chapter Six.

Headaches with direct dietary causes

Chinese Restaurant Syndrome
Chinese restaurants often add large amounts of monosodium glutamate (MSG), a common flavour enhancer, to the food they serve. MSG is also found in large amounts in soy sauce. It has a powerful effect on the blood vessels in the head, and can cause a very unpleasant headache. Anyone can suffer from this type of headache, not just migraine sufferers. However, some migraine sufferers find that they are especially vulnerable and that MSG can provoke an attack.

An MSG headache usually comes on about half an hour after eating a Chinese meal, and lasts for about an hour. There is pain in the forehead and a throbbing sensation in the temples. Some people are only affected if they eat MSG on an empty stomach.
MSG (additive E621) is also present in many packaged and processed foods, as it is a very popular flavour enhancer that is often used to improve the taste of poor-quality ingredients. The solution is either to check the labels of every tin and packet you eat, or to eat only fresh foods.

Processed meats headache
This is similar to Chinese Restaurant Syndrome, and is caused by the nitrates and nitrites used to preserve and colour processed meats. These, too, have an effect on the blood vessels, and can produce a throbbing headache if you are sensitive to them.
They are found in a wide range of processed meats, including hot dogs, salami, bacon, sausages and ham.

Ice cream headache
Some people find that eating very cold food, such as ice cream gives them a brief but sudden headache or toothache.

Hangovers
These happen because the blood vessels in the head are dilated (expanded) by the action of alcohol, a powerful vaso-active substance. As in a migraine attack, the expansion of the blood vessels causes the pain.

The worst offenders are red wine, cider, brandy, sherry and other alcoholic drinks that contain high levels of congeners. The least problematic are the 'pure' spirits like vodka and gin, and white wine. Some migraine sufferers are very sensitive to red wine. Some find that they can drink vintage red wine, but have to avoid the cheaper varieties.

Other types of headache
On occasion, headaches may prove to be a symptom of a more serious medical complaint – for example:

- eye problems (such as glaucoma)
- temporal arteritis
- brain tumours
- spinal problems
- dental problems
- high blood pressure
- injury
- infection
- sinusitis and catarrh
- hormonal problems.

If you suffer from regular or severe headaches, you must see your GP now. Problems such as brain tumours and meningitis are rare, but it makes no sense to take risks with your health.

Once the cause of your headaches has been identified and diagnosed, you will be free from worries about serious health problems, and can begin working towards a headache-free lifestyle.

Why do people get migraine?

Migraine isn't choosy: it affects both sexes, all ages and every walk of life. It does, however, follow certain identifiable patterns.

Children
Around 80 per cent of childhood sufferers are boys, although most adult sufferers are female. The peak incidence is around puberty and GCSEs – times of high stress.

Most children can and do grow out of migraine; although some will grow up to be adult migraine sufferers. They can be treated with drugs and relaxation therapy, and dietary therapy has also had some success in trials. Hypoglycaemia (low blood sugar) is also often a common problem.

Men
Men number about one-fifth of all adult migraineurs. Three-quarters of cluster headache sufferers are men.

Women
Around two-thirds of all migraine sufferers are women. In some, hormonal problems play a part, and stress and blood sugar problems are also important factors. Dietary therapy can be very useful, particularly in treating attacks that are menstrually-related.

The elderly
The great majority of migraine sufferers have developed the condition by the time they reach 40, and many find that their migraines disappear altogether in their later years. Again, though, nutrition has an important part to play. Elderly people on fixed incomes may not eat as well or as often as they need to, and this could precipitate attacks.

Migraine triggers

If you asked people in the street what they thought caused migraine, they would probably mention chocolate, cheese, stress and anxiety as some of the things that are most commonly associated with migraine attacks. But they would only be partly right as cheese, stress etc. are only a few of the trigger factors which can combine to produce an attack in a migraine sufferer.

Why we get migraine in the first place is a moot point. But it does seem that heredity has a part to play. At least 60 per cent of migraine sufferers seeking treatment have a close relative who is a sufferer. However, once that predisposition has been created, there still need to be triggers that spark off an attack.

Doctors now believe that there has to be a combination of triggers present in order for an attack to start. Some triggers, like stress and certain foods, are well known; but everyone's triggers are different. If you can identify and remove one or more of your personal trigger factors, then you may be able to stop having migraine attacks for good

Common triggers

Food and fasting
Some people know that certain foods; drinks or additives will trigger off a migraine attack. Others know that going without food for too long will have the same effect.

When I was a teenager, I used to get up late on a Saturday, eat very little breakfast, and go out shopping with friends. We were having so much fun that we stopped only for a bar of chocolate, before returning home for a very late lunch (often cheese). Every single Saturday evening, I had a terrible migraine attack. It didn't occur to me for ages that I was doing everything wrong.

By getting up late, I was getting too much sleep and depriving my body of food for longer than it was accustomed to. My blood sugar level was low and I was missing my morning 'fix' of coffee or tea. My tiny breakfast did little to raise my blood sugar level and I rushed about all morning, expending lots more energy and producing loads of adrenaline because I was excited and having fun after the stresses of a week's studying. The sugar in the bar of chocolate boosted my blood sugar level sky-high for a little while, after which it plummeted again. When I finally did get to eat something substantial it was cheese – a food well known for its migraine-inducing properties, as it is rich in tyramine, which has an effect on the blood vessels in the head.

Looking back, it's hardly surprising that I was ill every Saturday. At the time I put it down to relaxation after the working week, but the more I think about it, the more likely it seems that food – and the lack of food – contributed to my downfall.

Not everyone is sensitive to the typical 'migraine' foods (cheese, chocolate, oranges and red wine). The lack of food, or the wrong sort of food, can be just as important, as blood sugar swings are a common factor in migraine attacks. Eating a slice of sugary cake may boost your blood sugar in the short term, but your body may over compensate by producing too much insulin, dramatically lowering it again. Overdoing a slimming diet may also cause problems, as may strenuous exercise coupled with delayed meals.

You may find that you can eat a 'problem' food at some times and not at others. Some women find they can eat chocolate any time except just before a period. Just to complicate matters, some people can be sensitive to common foods that we eat in large quantities, often several times a day, such as wheat or milk, and this can make identifying them very difficult.

It's not just the foods, either – it's the things we put into them, the flavourings and preservatives, thickeners and colourings. For a small number of sufferers, these may be a genuine problem.

The good news is that, for many migraine sufferers, food isn't problem at all. No-one can tell you whether or not it is going to be a problem for you. But if you are determined and work through the various stages outlined in the next few chapters, you should be able to identify your own personal dietary triggers – if any exist. If you find that you don't have any, the freedom from worrying about everything you eat may just be enough to reduce the frequency of your attacks.

Smoking
This is definitely a factor in some headaches, especially cluster headaches. One study indicated that 53 per cent of migraine sufferers became migraine-free when they gave up smoking and other migraine triggers, whereas only 13 per cent of non-smokers became migraine-free when they gave up trigger foods.

Stress
You may find that you suffer from attacks not during periods of stress, but immediately afterwards. It's as though your body manages to cope until the crisis is over and then forces you to take a rest.

Many people find that they get attacks at the weekends, when they are relaxing after a long and hectic week. This can be exacerbated by too much sleep, a late breakfast and caffeine withdrawal symptoms.

You may also find that chronic stress causes recurrent attacks. After a while, your body can take no more and forces a sort of 'power-cut' on you.

Excitement

This is another form of stress. No matter how much you are enjoying yourself, you can still be experiencing stress, as you are producing lots of adrenaline. Once the 'high' is gone, you may have an attack. You need to plan ahead, learn to relax properly and eat a balanced diet. These preparations will help you to enjoy yourself without fear of unpleasant consequences later on.

Posture

If you have a bad back, shoulders or neck, this can give you a headache. Lots of us have bad posture without even realizing it, and sitting at VDUs all day is a notorious cause of postural problems. An osteopath, chiropractor, physiotherapist or teacher of the Alexander Technique may be able to advise – or ask your Health and Safety or union representative at work.

Sleep disturbance

Too much or too little sleep may bring on an attack. Try not to disrupt your routine, particularly if it means that you will eat late. Fasting for long periods lowers your blood sugar and makes you vulnerable to an attack. Getting up at your normal time may eliminate 'weekend' headaches.

Illness

You may find that your attacks are worse or more frequent when you are ill and at a low ebb.

Environmental factors

Many sufferers find that they are sensitive to bright light, flickering light, strong smells, stuffy atmospheres and fluorescent lighting. Some may find they cannot tolerate certain household chemicals.

Your personal triggers

As we have seen, migraine is a complex disorder and there are no easy answers. Each individual will have his or her own personal triggers, and it is only by identifying and – if possible – eliminating those triggers that the root cause of the problem can be addressed.

Not everyone is sensitive to individual foods, but most migraine sufferers will find that there is a dietary element to the incidence of their attacks, if only because of over-enthusiastic slimming, eating too much sugar, or exercising on an empty stomach. In the next few chapters, we will look at how to go about identifying your personal triggers and ways of using food to make you well rather than ill.

Chapter Two

Why watch your diet?

If your GP has diagnosed you as suffering from migraine, the chances are that he or she has also told you about some of the common migraine food triggers: chocolate, oranges, cheese, and red wine are the ones most people know about. They are often implicated as suspects because they contain vaso-active substances (chemicals that have an effect on the blood vessels, making them constrict or dilate).

It's certainly useful to keep an eye on these foods if they form part of your diet, but they aren't triggers for all migraine sufferers, and there may be others which seem more innocent but which are much more damaging to the individual sufferer's state of health. Some people can down a slice of chocolate orange cheesecake, washed down with a glass of Beaujolais Nouveau, without the slightest twinge. Others can't eat a slice of bread without feeling ill.

The problem is that each person reacts differently to different foods, and there are plenty of people who don't have any problems with food at all. In order to give the dietary approach some chance of working, you need to identify your own, personal triggers.

What's food got to do with it?

In the last chapter, we talked about triggers – factors, in our own lives and in the world around us, which may combine to increase the likelihood of a migraine attack.

Food is an important trigger, and identifying any dietary problems that you may have can make a significant difference to the quality of your life. The great thing about the dietary approach is that it's something that – with proper medical advice – you can do yourself. Perhaps for the first time since you began suffering from migraine, you can begin to feel that you are in control of your body, in control of your symptoms, in control of the way you feel.

The relationship between migraine and food is a complex one, and food can affect migraine sufferers in a variety of different ways.

Known migraine triggers

These are foods which contain substances known to trigger migraine attacks in some sufferers. Very important among these substances are the vaso-active amines, chemicals which have an effect on the blood vessels, making them constrict (narrow) or dilate (expand). As we saw in Chapter One, constriction and dilation of the blood vessels in the head are important features of migraine attacks.

Migraine attacks may not occur immediately after these foods are eaten: there can be a delay of up to 36 hours, until the point when the food has entered the liver and is being processed by enzymes. Doctors think that migraine sufferers may lack sufficient quantities of an enzyme called monoamine oxidase, which breaks down vaso-active amines and reduces their effect on the body.

Foods that contain vaso-active amines include:

- cheese: contains tyramine. Blue cheeses and matured cheeses contain the most. Cottage cheese, Philadelphia, cream cheese and quark contain no detectable tyramine;
- alcohol: contains histamine and is itself a vaso-active substance. Red wine, brandy, sherry are all bad. Gin and vodka may cause fewer problems because they contain few congeners;
- chocolate: contains phenylethylamine (dark chocolate is worse than milk or white);
- citrus fruits: contain synephrine. Watch out for foods that may contain traces of citrus, such as marmalade and flavourings. Concentrated juice tends to be the worst, because it contains the pips and skin, which have the highest concentration of synephrine and octopamine.

Other foods that are quite frequently cited as migraine 'culprits' include:

- pork
- bananas
- onions
- fish/seafood
- wheat

- fried food
- caffeine (found in coffee, tea, chocolate, cocoa, cola and some headache remedies)
- monosodium glutamate (E621)
- aspartame (sugar substitute) [but not saccharin]
- sodium benzoate (preservative)
- smoked foods
- dairy products

Fasting
As we have seen, doing without food can cause as many problems as eating the wrong foods. Simply sleeping in for an extra hour and/or going without breakfast may be enough to do the damage, particularly if you are relaxing after a busy week. Eating a diet high in junk food, with long gaps between irregular and poorly balanced meals, can cause problems with blood sugar levels. Fasting plus stress plus a trigger food will almost certainly add up to a migraine attack.

Additives and chemicals
Many food additives are natural substances, but others are man-made chemicals, added to food to preserve, flavour or colour it. Some of these may cause problems for migraine sufferers. Even natural substances can cause problems if they're one of your triggers. Don't assume that just because a label says 'natural' or 'healthy' it will necessarily be right for you. Monosodium glutamate (MSG) is a known culprit, as are nitrites and the nitrates sodium benzoate, sulphur dioxide and aspartame.

Related to this are problems with the environment around us household chemicals, smoke, fumes, perfumes, paint, moulds, dust mites, cavity wall insulation, and even the smell of warm plastic, which can trigger attacks in some people. It is well worth identifying and addressing any environmental triggers as well as dietary ones.

Food allergy
Food allergy is the reaction of the body's immune system, reacting to the invasion of a foreign protein – true food allergy is quite rare, and can be serious. for example milk, peanuts or wheat. At its most extreme the reaction can be life-threatening anaphylactic shock, in

which the sufferer's lips, tongue and throat may swell up, impeding breathing.

If you have a fixed allergy, you will react each time you encounter a problem substance, however small the amount. If you have a variable allergy, it is harder for doctors to identify as it depends on the amount taken, and the response to it may vary. Sometimes the response may be delayed, or there may be no response at all.

Food sensitivity

This is believed to be much more common than food allergy, and many experts feel it is an important element in many migraine attacks.

Food sensitivity is also referred to as 'food intolerance', or 'maladaptation syndrome'. It isn't an immune reaction, producing antibodies, so many doctors would disagree with defining it as an allergic reaction – although some experts do use the terms 'allergy' and 'intolerance' interchangeably. Reactions can be subtle, delayed and/or masked, so it can be quite difficult to link a culprit food with its reaction.

Food sensitivity or intolerance can be defined as an abnormal reaction to a substance that most people can tolerate without difficulty. For example, milk allergy is rare, but it has been estimated that up to 70 per cent of people worldwide may have some degree of intolerance (sensitivity) to cow's milk.

It has been suggested that around one in ten of all migraine sufferers have some sort of 'food sensitivity'. In other words, their bodies refuse to tolerate certain foods which other people can consume without problems. In some cases these are single foods; in other cases (some would say more frequently), the sufferer will have multiple food sensitivities. This can make them all the more difficult to track down, because you may need to eliminate all the culprit foods before you begin to feel better.

In many cases the 'culprit' foods will not be the typical migraine triggers of cheese, red wine, citrus fruits and so on, but quite ordinary foods which we eat often and don't associate with bad reactions, because these reactions are delayed or masked. Apparently innocent foods like wheat, milk, yeast and chicken have frequently been found to cause problems, and it is possible to be intolerant to just about anything – especially if you eat a lot of it.

There is evidence to suggest that eating too much of any one food may make you prone to developing a sensitivity to that food.

Does food intolerance really exist?

There is still some doubt among conventional medical practitioners about the extent of food intolerance as a problem. Indeed, a minority of doctors still dispute its existence.

Whilst it is certainly true that dietary problems can be imagined, or exacerbated by anxiety bordering on obsession, most experts agree that food sensitivities can cause problems for some migraine sufferers.

One theory put forward is that the plants we regard as our natural food were not specifically designed to be eaten by humans. Some contain toxins which exist to protect the plant from predators. When we eat them, we have to detoxify these chemicals in our livers.

This process works well when we are omnivorous and don't eat much of any one thing, but our modern diet has come to rely upon certain 'staple' foods, like wheat and milk. These are the two most frequently eaten foods in the West, and they are also the two most common culprits in food intolerance. Interestingly, in countries that have different diets, the incidence of intolerances is also different: e.g. rice and soya are the most prevalent intolerances in the Far East.

By eating large amounts of one food, the experts tell us, we run the risk of developing intolerance to that food. If you stop eating a 'culprit' food for a while, the intolerance may be reduced; but if you start eating it again regularly the symptoms are likely to return with a vengeance. So, the experts say, in order to promote good health we should try to eat as varied a diet as possible.

What do the scientists say?

Scientific opinion remains divided about the nature and extent of food intolerance. However, the scientific trials which have been carried out would seem to suggest that food intolerance does play a significant role in many cases of migraine.

Charing Cross Hospital

Trials were carried out on 60 patients during 1979. Of the 60 patients tested, 85 per cent became migraine-free after their food intolerances had been identified.

Great Ormond Street Children's Hospital

Between 1982 and 1983, clinical trials were carried out at Great Ormond Street Children's Hospital. Interestingly, four out of the five doctors who conducted the trials had grave reservations about the role of food intolerance in migraine.

Eighty-eight children took part in the trials, all of them sufferers from frequent, severe migraine attacks. Over two-thirds of them also suffered from digestive symptoms such as diarrhoea, flatulence and abdominal pain. Other symptoms reported included runny or blocked noses, aching limbs, epileptic fits, mouth ulcers, vaginal discharge, asthma and eczema.

The children were asked to follow a simple diet consisting of one type of meat, one fruit, one vegetable and either rice or potatoes. They were given vitamin and calcium supplements to compensate for any nutritional deficiencies, and stayed on the diet for three or four weeks.

When children experienced an improvement in their symptoms certain foods were reintroduced into their diet. If these foods caused symptoms they were withdrawn again. Later, when all common foods had been tried, each child was tested again, with one of the foods that had caused a severe reaction. This test was conducted double-blind, so that even the doctors conducting the trials did not know which children had been given suspect foods, and which were given a placebo. Out of 40 children, 35 were made ill by the suspect food and only two by the placebo.

Seventy-eight of the 88 children recovered completely on a simple diet, and only six showed no improvement. In 74 cases, particular foods could be identified as triggers, and were eliminated.

Fitzsimons Army Medical Center, Colorado

A group of 104 patients were asked to eliminate wheat, corn, milk, eggs and any foods to which they reacted in a skin-prick allergy test. Two-thirds improved, and 38 per cent had a better than 50 per cent reduction in their migraine attacks.

University of Texas

Skin-prick tests were given to 43 adult migraine sufferers. If positive reactions were produced, the relevant foods were eliminated. Those who had no positive reactions were put on a diet free from wheat, corn, milk and eggs. Thirty per cent had fewer migraines, and 70 per cent of these responded in a double-blind test.

Are you food-sensitive?

It isn't always easy to tell which foods are your own personal 'culprits'. This is because, unlike food allergy, the results of food sensitivity can take time to appear. If, for example, you are sensitive to raspberries and to milk, and you eat a slice of raspberry Pavlova, the migraine attack (or other symptoms) might take 36 hours or longer to develop. Even then, you can't be sure if it was the raspberries or the cream, or both, which caused your attack.

Food addiction

To make matters even more complicated, the foods which make you ill can also be the ones which make you feel better … for a little while. When you stop eating them, you may suffer from bad withdrawal symptoms which prompt you to get another 'fix' of the food which you think makes you feel better, because it relieves your symptoms.

Of course, it is this very food which has made you feel unwell in the first place.

When you crave the very foods which make you ill, this is referred to as food addiction. It is a form of hidden or masked food intolerance.

Hidden intolerance

This is also known as 'masked' intolerance or sensitivity. It was first described by the famous allergist Dr Herbert Rinkel.

According to this curious mechanism, a food can make you ill without your realizing it. It's quite likely to be a food you eat frequently, maybe several times a day, and although your body is sensitive to it, the reaction becomes damped down over a period of time, as you accustom yourself to regular doses of the food.

The symptoms of intolerance may not always be the ones you might expect. For example, eating something you're sensitive to won't necessarily give you abdominal problems or a headache. Rinkel discovered that his permanently runny nose was in fact allergic rhinitis, caused by eating too many eggs.

An acute reaction to the food may flare up from time to time, particularly if other trigger factors such as stress, excitement or disturbed sleep patterns are present. In some cases, when the intolerance has gone on for a long time but the food is still eaten regularly, the body reaches a stage where it can no longer cope, and when resistance runs out serious and debilitating symptoms can occur.

Like food addiction, this can be difficult to deal with. If you stop eating the food you may experience severe withdrawal symptoms at first, driving you back to eating the trigger food. After an extra hour or two of sleep, you may wake up with the beginnings of a migraine attack, the result of missing out on your regular dose of 'culprit' food.

Threshold dose
The threshold dose is the amount of a food (or other substance) which you need to consume in order to produce a reaction. You may be able to eat small amounts of trigger foods without having a migraine attack, but if you eat the trigger food several times in short succession, or at certain times of the month (e.g. just before a period), this may be enough to make you ill.

The apparent inconsistency of the reaction may make it difficult to work out which foods are actually at fault, particularly if you have multiple sensitivities. Two or more trigger foods may combine to push you over the threshold dose and give you a headache, migraine attack or other symptoms.

Chemical sensitivity
This is often related to food sensitivity, and it is easy to confuse intolerance to a food with intolerance to a chemical. For example, you may not be sensitive to apples, but to the paraffin wax they are coated with to improve their shelf-life. Similarly, bananas are ripened with ethylene gas, and corn (maize) is soaked in sulphur dioxide to stop fermentation. Eating organic products helps to

isolate this type of related sensitivity.

Be aware of other 'allergens' which may be present in your home and work environment: air pollution, cigarette smoke, solvents, perfumes, plastics and so on. All of these may cause adverse reactions in a small number of people.

The signs of food sensitivity

Headaches and migraine are one aspect of the broad spectrum of symptoms associated with food, chemical and environmental sensitivities. The following is not an exhaustive list, but it will give you some idea of the wide range of conditions and symptoms which have been interpreted as indicators of food sensitivity:

- weight problems; being consistently over or underweight
- persistent fatigue
- swelling (eyes, hands, abdomen, ankles) and fluid retention
- recurrent mouth ulcers
- aching muscles
- joint pain, rheumatoid arthritis
- palpitations, rapid heart rate after meals
- sweating
- feeling ill on waking
- headaches and migraine
- mental problems – e.g. depression, anxiety, hyperactivity in children
- digesting problems – e.g. bloating, diarrhoea, vomiting, nausea, stomach and duodenal ulcers, irritable bowel syndrome, constipation, flatulence, Crohn's disease, coeliac disease (a lifelong intolerance to wheat)
- general malaise

If you suffer from one or more of these symptoms, this does not necessarily mean that you suffer from food intolerance, but it is certainly worth working through the regimes recommended in the next two chapters. You may discover that you have sensitivities you had never suspected. Alternatively, you may free yourself from the worry that you are eating foods that are making you ill.

What can be done about food sensitivity?

Each migraine sufferer has different triggers. In many cases these will not include food triggers, and for some people the task of identifying triggers is a simple one. But at the other end of the spectrum some sufferers experience multiple sensitivities which can only be identified using a logical and systematic approach.

The system recommended by most doctors and nutritionists is the exclusion or elimination diet, which has been used in a variety of clinical trials and demonstrated to be effective. Over the next two chapters, we will be looking at the best way to go about identifying your own food triggers using this technique.

What are the benefits?

Getting rid of any trigger is a good idea for the migraine sufferer for, as we have seen, it takes a combination of factors to set off an attack. Removing just one of these players from the arena may make all the difference, and eliminate – or at the very least reduce the frequency of – your attacks.

If, when you have worked your way through this book, you come to the conclusion that you don't have any food sensitivities, that too is a cause for celebration – never again will you have to turn down that cheese sandwich or that glass of Buck's Fizz! At the very least, this book should help you to devise a healthy eating programme that will increase your all-round health and wellbeing.

The dietary approach: what's in it for you?
You can expect to derive at least some of the following benefits if you invest time and determination in the dietary approach.

- Your improved general health will improve as a result through sensible, balanced eating, thinking about what you're putting into your body and making sure it has everything it needs.
- You will experience psychological benefits: you're doing something to help yourself, taking control of an illness which can so easily take over your life. A greater sense of wellbeing should result.

- Eating the right things regularly helps to stabilize blood sugar levels, staving off hypoglycaemia and all the problems that go with it (mood-swings, migraines, sensitivity to cold and so on).
- You may be able to identify and eliminate an existing nutritional deficiency;
- You may lose (or gain) weight.
- You may reduce the frequency and/or severity of your migraine attacks.
- You may also help to reduce the frequency and/or severity of other types of headache.

Chapter Three

Finding your food triggers (I)

In the last chapter, we looked at the different ways in which food – or the lack of it – can affect our bodies and help to trigger a migraine attack.

It has been suggested that some degree of food sensitivity (intolerance) is implicated in many cases of migraine, and it is definitely worth investing time and effort in finding out if you have any food allergies, sensitivities or triggers.

The chances are that if you have a food allergy, you will already know about it, as the symptoms tend to manifest themselves rapidly and can be quite dramatic, ranging from swelling, tingling, wheezing and hives (a raised red rash) to anaphylactic shock in the most extreme cases.

Food intolerance, on the other hand, is much harder to identify, and doctors, nutritionists and other experts have spent many years trying to develop the perfect test. At the time of writing, there is still no procedure that is both quick and 100 per cent reliable.

However, a wide range of tests are available, and it is a good idea to be aware of them in case you see them advertised in the press, or are offered them by a doctor or alternative practitioner. You can then weigh up the pros and cons for yourself, and decide whether or not you think they are worth a try.

Tests currently available to identify food intolerance

Prick and patch testing
This is the traditional test for allergies such as hay fever and allergic rhinitis (a runny or blocked-up nose) caused by an allergy to the household dust-mite. It was not designed as a test for food intolerance, but it has been adapted for use in this field.

In prick testing, a drop of fluid (the test reagent) is placed on the skin (usually the skin of the forearm), which is then pricked or scratched. The liquid contains a small amount of the substance to which the sufferer is thought to be sensitive. Often, several foods are tested at the same time, using separate drops of fluid. The patient is asked to wait for a given length of time (say, half an hour). If a raised weal is produced, this suggests an allergic reaction: the size of the weal indicates the strength of the reaction.

Patch testing is similar, using small amounts of the food taped to the forearm and left for a number of hours. In this case, reddening of the skin indicates the presence of an allergic reaction. A 'control' patch is also taped to the skin so that the tester can spot any reaction to the tape or pad used.

Advantages: cheap, not disruptive or invasive, unlikely to be any unpleasant side-effects.

Disadvantages: rather unreliable. There are said to be a lot of false negatives, so many sensitivities may not be picked up. Prick testing works quite well for airborne allergens like pollen and dust, but has not proved as successful as a test for food intolerance. Patch testing seems to work best for 'contact dermatitis' caused by a sensitivity to certain metals, detergents and the like.

The RAST (radioallergosorbent) test
This test is designed to measure antibodies in an individual's blood, produced in response to 'foreign' proteins such as pollen, dust or certain foods.

A food extract is applied to beads made from an inert substance. Then a sample of the sufferer's blood serum is brought into contact with the beads. Any antibodies produced will stick to the food antigens on the beads. The beads are then rinsed so that only the antibodies remain. Using a type of radioactive marker, it is possible to work out the amount of antibodies present in the patient's blood.

Advantages: no special advantages.

Disadvantages: expensive, complicated and not very reliable. Can produce false positives.

The cytotoxic test
This type of test has become very popular recently, as it has

received a great deal of publicity in the media. Advertisements are often aimed at failed dieters, who feel that their weight problems may derive from food intolerance.

A blood sample is taken from the sufferer and the white cells are removed. These white cells are tested by being exposed to a wide variety of substances, including common foods and chemicals.

The theory behind this test is that, if a sensitivity exists, the white cells will be damaged and may be killed. In severe cases, the cells may swell up and rupture. The reactions are observed in the laboratory and graded from 0 (no reaction at all) to 3 (a severe reaction).

The sufferer is then given a 'green' list of foods (which can be eaten safely), and a 'red' list (which should be avoided completely).

Advantages: this test only takes a few minutes and is relatively simple. Some dramatic successes have been claimed, not only with migraine patients but also with sufferers from other disorders, including obesity. It can be helpful in suggesting suspect foods that could be eliminated from the diet, or in confirming a sufferer's suspicions about foods which may be causing attacks.

Disadvantages: this is not a particularly accurate test, as recent investigations have proved. A Sunday newspaper recently asked a number of volunteers each to send two identical samples of their blood to a lab, each using two different names. The lab came up with widely differing results for identical blood samples. The Consumers' Association tried a similar experiment, using a woman who suffered from coeliac disease. The laboratory failed to identify any degree of wheat intolerance.

Many scientists feel that the technique used for identifying reactions is too subjective, relying upon observation rather than any absolute scientific standards. It has been claimed that laboratories often give inadequate advice when they send out the test results, and frequently fail to mention that the results only offer a picture of the sufferer's intolerances at one moment in time. The picture can change quickly, and in a few weeks or months the results might be significantly different.

The cytotoxic test is also expensive. It can cost between £100 and £200, with no guarantee of a satisfactory result.

Applied kinesiology
According to acupuncture and chiropractic, when the body is subjected to adverse influences certain muscles become weaker. A trained practitioner can detect these weaknesses and so diagnose food intolerance.

One technique is to put a sample of a suspect food under the sufferer's tongue, and then test the strength of the muscles to determine whether or not there is a sensitivity to that food. Weakening of the muscles suggests intolerance. Other practitioners claim that they can detect this weakening simply by giving the patient a sample or container of the food to hold.

Advantages: very cheap and quick, with no risk to the patient.

Disadvantages: each food has to be tested separately. The accuracy of the method is not known: it depends to some extent upon the skill and experience of the practitioner. Some successes claimed.

Vega testing
This technique – a sort of high-tech dowsing – was developed in Germany, and uses a Vega testing machine to detect food intolerance. Solutions of different substances are put into the machine and the patient is given an electrode to hold, whilst the practitioner touches different points on the patient's body with a metal probe. Any reaction is registered by a needle on a dial.

Advantages: said to be useful for detecting all sorts of 'energy imbalances' in the body.

Disadvantages: as yet not entirely accurate, but offers promise for further development.

Dowsing
This is sometimes (incorrectly) referred to as 'hair analysis'.
A lock of the patient's hair is given or sent to the practitioner, and a pendulum is swung over it. It is said to move differently if allergy or intolerance is present.

Advantages: non-invasive, no risk to patient, patient does not need to be present during the test.

Disadvantages: can be expensive, no evidence at all that it works, practitioners need not be trained or regulated.

Hair analysis
A sample of hair is taken from the patient and analysed for its vitamin, mineral, protein content and so on.

Advantages: non-invasive, no risk to patient, patient does not need to be present during test.

Disadvantages: no evidence that it is of any value in food intolerance/allergy, though it may help to pinpoint nutritional deficiencies. Can be expensive and practitioners may be untrained.

Auriculo-cardiac reflex (ACR)
ACR was developed at the University of Southampton's Centre for the Study of Complementary Medicine. It involves measuring movement in the point of maximum amplitude in the pulse (reflex) in response to stimulation. Filters containing each substance are held over the skin and the reflex measured.

Advantages: non-invasive, quick, claimed to be moderately successful.

Disadvantages: rather hit-and-miss, requires highly trained and skilled practitioners, not wholly reliable.

To test or not to test?

As we have seen, some of the tests currently available to diagnose food intolerance are little more than magical mumbo-jumbo, whilst even the most scientifically respected tests do not claim anything like 100 per cent success.

None of the tests described above is likely to do you any harm (though you should discuss them with your doctor before going ahead, particularly if a blood test is involved). They may even provide a starting point as you set out to identify your own food sensitivities, perhaps jogging your memory about foods which may have made you ill in the past.

On the other hand, they may do you no good at all, and some of them will certainly set you back a bit financially. Whether or not you opt for testing is your decision. If you do, and if you can afford it, it may be a good idea to try several different methods, and compare the results that they produce. Is there any agreement on what is making you ill? Or have you been presented with a whole host of conflicting facts that leave you even more confused than you were before?

If you do find the same foods mentioned consistently, make a careful note of them and consider them as prime suspects. They will be a useful starting point when you begin excluding possible culprit foods from your diet.

Keeping a migraine diary

You will be familiar with the concept of a migraine diary. It is the most reliable and systematic way in which you can begin to identify your personal migraine triggers, including any possible problems with food tolerance.

Best of all, keeping a migraine diary costs virtually nothing! The only cost (apart from paper and a pen) is in time, commitment, organization and determination: if you want it to work, you must persevere, filling in the details for each category every day, and omitting nothing.

In order for your diary to work as a diagnostic tool it must be complete, so that any recurring patterns are clearly revealed. You must make up your mind, at the outset, that you will fill in everything as it happens, or as soon afterwards as is humanly possible. It's no use waiting a week and then trying to fill the details in from memory: can you really remember if you ate cabbage for dinner last Thursday? Your diary must become a daily task.

A migraine diary is of use not just to you, as the sufferer, but to your GP and to any practitioner who helps you with your migraine. It provides a meticulous record of all your attacks, your diet, your sleep patterns . . . in short, a complete picture of you and the way you live.

It will help you to discover not only any food intolerance problems, but the other triggers which combine to produce your attacks: stress, disturbed sleep patterns, fasting, climate, chemical sensitivities and so on. Knocking out one or more of these triggers may be enough to reduce or eliminate your attacks.

Creating your own migraine diary

What should it look like?

Remember: your migraine diary is there to help you, and it should be as user-friendly as possible. The easier it is to use, the more inclined you will be to make regular use of it. Also, it needs to be set out clearly, as you (and quite possibly your doctor) will be referring to it later on, using it to identify patterns in your migraine attacks.

Opt for a large format: one A4 'Landscape' sheet per page is nice and roomy. You will need to fit lots of information onto each page, so you don't want it to be cramped and difficult to read. Some people like to use an exercise book or desk diary, ruled into columns. Others prefer to draw up one diary page on a sheet of plain A4 paper, then make photocopies and keep them in a loose-leaf file. The best place for your migraine diary is in the kitchen. Since, for the time being, you are primarily interested in food and the effect it is having on your body, it makes sense to keep your diary right next to the food. That way, you will have no excuse for not noting down everything you eat, including every midnight trip to the fridge!

One last word of advice: keep a pen by the diary at all times and don't let anyone else walk off with it!

What information should you include?

The layout of your diary is up to you, but it needs to be clear and uncluttered. Because your migraine diary contains lots of additional information about food and drink, it will take up a lot of space. You may find it helpful to use two pages per day: one for details of your attacks, and one for food and other possible triggers (e.g. extra stress, missed meals, travel). The information which you need to include is as follows:

- month, date, day, time of day
- daily details of pain – not just migraine attacks but other headaches too (is the pain mild, moderate, severe?)
- time and duration of any attacks
- any nausea and/or vomiting
- any medication taken (prescription and over-the-counter remedies, including remedies from health-food stores), with time taken
- any home remedies and strategies (hot water bottles, glasses of water, cold compresses and so on)
- menstruation
- all food eaten, with rough amounts and times eaten
- all drink taken, with rough amounts and times drunk
- any missed or delayed meals, or start of a slimming diet
- any additional travel
- any additional stress, or busy day at work, excitement, or sudden news
- any additional exercise (e.g. sport)
- bowel movements (especially unusual, loose, painful or constipated)
- any change to normal sleeping patterns (including sleeping late).

Don't forget that drinks and medicines (both prescribed and non-prescribed) also count in your food diary, because they are substances that you take into your body. Below is a sample layout for a migraine diary. It is only intended as a guideline, and you can vary the layout to suit yourself. But remember to include all the information suggested: an incomplete record may not be sufficient to identify all your triggers.

Saturday 6 March

	7.30am	1.00pm	2.00pm	10.00pm	Midnight
Food	Porridge, toast marmalade, sugar	Cheese sandwich pickle, sponge cake	Club biscuit	Chicken vindaloo rice, raita nan, onion bhaji	
Drink	Tea with milk, 2 cups	Can of Coke	Orange fizzy crink	2 pints of lager, 1 cup Expresso coffee	Coffee
Stress?	Feeling relaxed after busy week. Excited about tonight's birthday party at Indian restaurant				
Exercise			Roller skating at rink		
Sleep	Normal				Got to bed very late — 1.00pm
Menstruation	Some PMS symptoms. Sore breasts				

Sunday 7 March

	10.00am	2.30pm	4.00pm	6.00pm	6.00pm onwards
Food	croissants (2) butter, jam	roast lamb new potatoes peas, mint sauce, stewed rhubarb & custard	peppermint teas		plain tap water sips
Drink	brewed coffee 3 cups	red wine (half bottle)			
Stress	In-laws coming over for lunch	Rowed with in-laws about the kids			
Exercise	Dug garden (am)				
Sleep	got to bed late, disturbed night, overslept			went to bed at 6.00pm	managed to get to sleep around 11.00pm

Attack Diary : sample page

Saturday and Sunday

March	Pain	When Started	Duration	Nausea/ Vomiting	Medication	When Taken	Home Remedies/ Strategies
Sat. 6	mild	6.00pm	3 hours	no	2 aspirin	7pm	—
Sun. 7	severe	4.00pm	until went to sleep (late at night)	yes	too sick	—	peppermint tea and hot water bottle

Analysing the results

Follow your diary for a month at least – several months if your migraine attacks are fairly widely spaced. It may take time for patterns to emerge if you only suffer from attacks, say once or twice a month.

Once you are satisfied that you have a complete record, sit down and try to identify any possible triggers. There are a number of questions which you will need to ask yourself:

- Are there any specific foods that you feel may be responsible for triggering your attacks? Make a note of any you suspect.
- Do you think the 'typical' migraine-inducers – citrus, cheese. chocolate and red wine – have any affect on your attacks? If so, vaso-active amines may be a problem.
- Do any foods, drinks, medicines and such like seem to have been consumed consistently up to 36 hours before an attack? Note them down.
- Do your attacks seem to follow a period of fasting: a missed meal, a late breakfast etc? If so, low blood sugar could be a factor in your attacks.

- Do you get an attack after strenuous exercise? Again, low blood sugar could be implicated.
- Do your attacks seem to come after eating a lot of sugary or highly processed, 'fast' foods? Violent swings in blood sugar levels may be to blame. Also, additives such as MSG may have an effect upon the blood vessels, triggering an attack.

These are just a few of the questions which can help you to identify the culprit foods which may be making you ill. In the next chapter, we shall be looking at some of the most common culprits, and how you can use elimination dieting to identify those which may be a problem for you.

Chapter Four

Finding your food triggers (II)

Now that you have been keeping a migraine diary for several weeks or months, you may be starting to identify possible trigger foods. Keep a note of these, as you will be testing them to see if they do in fact cause you problems.

Elimination diets

Elimination (or exclusion) diets are the most reliable method of pinpointing your food triggers in a controlled and systematic way. They will help you to identify foods to which you have developed an intolerance as well as and foods that affect you because they contain migraine-inducing substances, such as tyramine.

The basic principle is a simple one. In order to find out whether or not a food is triggering your migraine attacks, it needs to be eliminated from your diet. However, simply removing a single food from your diet may not be enough to make you feel better. One reason for this is that some people have multiple sensitivities. If you are one of these people, it may not be until all of the culprit foods are removed that you begin to show an improvement.

There are two phases to a typical elimination diet:

Exclusion

In this phase, the suspect food is eliminated completely for up to three weeks. This allows time for all traces to be removed from the body.

At first, you may feel much worse, as you begin to suffer 'withdrawal symptoms' and crave the very food which has been making you ill. If you have an intolerance to the food (and if all of your problem foods have been eliminated), you should feel much better by the end of the first week. You are then ready to reintroduce the foods, one by one, until you discover which ones have been making you ill.

Challenging

After approximately three weeks, challenge-testing takes place. This involves reintroducing the food, eating it in moderate quantities over two or three meals, and waiting to see if there are any adverse reactions. A migraine attack can take up to 36 hours to develop, so you need to wait this long to be sure that side effects aren't going to appear. Three weeks is the longest that you should wait before challenge-testing, if you wait too long food sensitivity can die down and it takes time to build up again: it is difficult to spot the reaction when you re-introduce the culprit food.

After the elimination diet

If you do confirm that you have a sensitivity to a particular food, you will need to eliminate it from your diet and find a suitably nutritious alternative. Food sensitivities can and do change with time, so it is worth repeating the challenge test after six months. If there are no adverse symptoms, you can reintroduce the food to your diet. But you must eat it with caution, and must not slip into the pattern of eating it more often than once every fourth or fifth day, as you risk redeveloping the old intolerance problem.

If, after a six-monthly and twelve-monthly challenge, you find that you are still intolerant to the food, it is best to eliminate it permanently from your diet.

Common culprits

As we have seen, in theory just about any food can cause problems for the migraine sufferer, for one of several reasons:

- It contains vaso-active substances (eg cheese, citrus fruits, monosodium glutamate). Not every migraine sufferer reacts badly to these substances, so it is important to test them rather than simply cutting them out of your diet – particularly as some of them have a high nutritional value.
- You have developed an intolerance to it (a particular problem with foods we eat a great deal of).
- You are not eating properly, and your blood sugar levels are uncontrolled (eg you eat a lot of sugar-rich junk food, salt, caffeine or refined carbohydrates).
- It contains additives to which you have become sensitive (eg tartrazine, aspartame).

Below, some of the foods most commonly implicated in migraine are listed. It certainly doesn't claim to be an exhaustive list, but it may help you to draw up your own list of 'prime suspects'. It's worth bearing in mind that the foods that cause intolerance problems are frequently:

- those we crave or like best
- those we have disliked since childhood, but eat dutifully because 'they do us good'
- those we eat every day, and which form a staple part of the standard Western diet (e.g. wheat, milk).
- It is highly unlikely that you will be sensitive to more than a few of these substances, and you must not on any account cut out large numbers of foods from your diet without:
- following a properly devised elimination diet incorporating suitable alternative foods
- doing so under medical supervision.
- You should also be careful never to follow an elimination diet for more than three weeks at a time (three to five days in the case of a fast). After this time, you must begin reintroducing foods, not only to challenge-test but also to increase the nutritional value of your diet.
- Foods known to have vaso-active effects
- chocolate (especially dark)
- cheese (except cream, cottage, quark, Philadelphia, curd)
- citrus fruit (lime, lemon, orange, grapefruit, ugli, mandarin and so on)
- bananas (especially ripe)
- seafood
- monosodium glutamate
- nitrites and nitrates (in preserved meats)
- caffeine (coffee, tea, cola, cocoa, chocolate)
- alcohol
- dates
- raspberries
- avocados
- olives
- smoked fish and other smoked foods,

Foods known to cause intolerance problems in some adults

- wheat
- milk
- instant coffee
- yeast
- cheese
- sugar
- citrus fruit
- tea
- tomatoes
- fish
- fried foods
- grapes
- soya
- nuts (especially peanuts, walnuts)
- oats
- egg
- beef
- corn
- chocolate
- onions
- pork
- potato
- peaches
- chicken
- strawberries
- melons
- carrots
- pickles and vinegar
- liquorice.

Additives which may cause problems for migraine sufferers

- monosodium glutamate (flavour enhancer E621)
- aspartame (hut not saccharin)
- nitrites and nitrates
- sodium benzoate/benzoic acid
- tartrazine (colouring El 02)

- sulphur dioxide (used to treat dried fruit and in processed foods)
- salt.

Medicines

Remember that medicines, too, can contain problem ingredients, for example:

- many over-the-counter pain-relievers contain caffeine
- many syrup-based products, such as cough linctus, contain colourings and sugar
- some decongestants mimics the effects of adrenaline

The least common culprits

As we have said, just about any food can be a problem food which is why we must all search out and identify our own food triggers. There are no such things as universal good guys and bad guys. But, just as there are common culprits, there are also a number of foods that are rarely implicated in migraine. If you are pretty sure they are not triggers for you, you might consider using them as the basis of an elimination diet, as they are fairly unlikely to cause a reaction.

If, after the first week, you experience no improvement or a worsening of your symptoms, you will need to try a different elimination diet – ideally, one based upon foods which you rarely eat such as mango, kiwi fruit, venison, millet (an 'exotic' or 'rare' foods diet). Many experts believe that foods you have rarely eaten are unlikely to be culprits in food sensitivity.

Reasonably 'safe' foods, from an intolerance point of view, are:

- lamb, turkey
- pears, unsweetened pear juice
- brussel sprouts, courgettes, cauliflower, carrots, broccoli.

However, it is best to begin gradually, as few people will need to follow such a strict regime.

Preparing for your elimination diet

Before starting the first phase of your diet, there are several steps that

51

you should take.

- Keep a migraine/food diary for at least one month, preferably longer, and take a note of all the foods which you consider 'suspect'.
- Give up smoking. Many migraine sufferers have reported an impressive reduction in the frequency and severity of their attacks on giving up smoking. Nicotine, like caffeine, is a stimulant and the end result is likely to be more adrenaline, more migraines. Smoking also hinders the absorption of essential nutrients, and giving up will help to free your body from toxins and improve your general health and resistance.
- Don't plan your diet for a busy or stressful time. Aim to fit it in at a time when you don't have a lot of work or social commitments.
- Plan ahead. Buy in food for the first couple of weeks, and plan your menus, packed lunches and so on, so that you don't have to agonize about what to eat and you aren't tempted to cheat. Even one tiny cheat will undo all the good you have done, and you will have to start all over again, from the beginning!
- If you know you are going to have to eat out, warn your host/ess in advance. In restaurants, choose plain, fresh foods and if you're avoiding caffeine, take herbal tea bags or stick to mineral water.
- Pre-cook and freeze meals in bulk.
- See your GP and put him/her in the picture. Discuss whether or not there are any medical reasons why you should not take part in an elimination diet (e.g. diabetes). You may also discuss whether or not it is possible to give up any prescription drugs you are taking, without undesirable side effects. Never stop taking prescription drugs without your doctor's full support. It could be dangerous.
- If you are taking the oral contraceptive pill, ask your doctor if it would be feasible to stop taking it for the duration of your elimination diet. Some migraine sufferers find that taking the Pill increases the frequency and severity of their attacks.
- Make sure, though, that you and your partner are using a satisfactory alternative form of contraception.
- Consider taking a nutritional supplement if you think your diet may be deficient. If you eat a lot of wheat bran, it is possible you may not be getting enough calcium, zinc, iron and magnesium, as

a substance called phytate can impair their absorption. (There is no need to worry about wholemeal bread, as yeast breaks down phytates.) It is possible that you have other nutritional deficiencies, too. But avoid food supplements which contain colourings and flavourings; some health-food shops now stock 'hypo-allergenic' brands.

- Avoid processed, tinned, packaged and prepared foods. Although foods have to be labelled nowadays, it isn't always easy to tell what's in them, as additives go under a variety of baffling technical names.
- If you can, persuade your family to go on the diet with you. This will make life easier for you, and reduce temptation. You may also find that one or more of the other family members benefits from the diet too, as food intolerance is thought to run in families.

Never put a child on any sort of diet without medical approval. Elimination diets for children are discussed in Chapter Eight.

The elimination diet

Phase 1: eating healthily, eating well
The first step to take is to ensure that you are eating a balanced, healthy diet. It's surprising how many of us are just too busy and overstressed to eat properly. In fact, some problems which are thought to be caused by food intolerance are in fact the result of poor nutrition and dietary deficiencies. A lack of essential vitamins, minerals and fatty acids can produce a variety of unwelcome symptoms and will reduce your resistance to stress and problem foods.

If you feel you need one, take a food supplement. But ideally, it is best to get all your nutrients from good, healthy, fresh food, which should supply all that your body needs. Eating healthily is a good habit to get into.

Do plan ahead, and don't have lots of 'banned' foods tucked away at the back of your kitchen cupboards, just waiting for you to yield to temptation. Make sure you have an ample supply of nutritious snacks for when you feel like that bar of chocolate or that bag of crisps.
'Banned' food

- chocolate, cocoa, cola drinks
- processed meats e.g. bacon, corned beef, sausages, salami
- smoked foods
- ripe cheeses
- artificial sweeteners
- colourings, preservatives, flavourings, antioxidants, stabilizers etc (if in doubt, avoid all E numbers)
- spicy foods e.g. curries, chilli
- fast food and takeaways
- alcohol
- margarine
- pies
- fish fingers
- wheat bran
- highly-salted foods
- coffee and tea (cut out slowly, to avoid withdrawal symptoms)
- sugar and sugary foods
- aspirin
- painkillers containing caffeine
- medicines which contain colourings.

In addition to the above, you should also eliminate any suspect foods identified by your migraine diary, or by other forms of testing. You may wish to cut out citrus fruits as well.

Foods allowed on the diet

- fresh fruit and vegetables (except suspects, such as citrus fruits)
- fresh meat and fish
- wholemeal bread
- milk
- butter
- cheeses which are low in tyramine (e.g. cream cheese)
- wholewheat breakfast cereals
- rice
- beans and pulses, lentils
- pastry (if home-made, preferably with wholemeal flour)
- fruit juice (fresh and unsweetened).

What to watch out for

If you feel worse initially, don't panic. You may be suffering from caffeine withdrawal symptoms, or withdrawal from a food to which you are intolerant. If the symptoms persist after the first week on the diet, you may be intolerant to one or more of the foods you are still eating; and you will need to move on to the next phase – the basic elimination diet.

If you feel better after the first few days, you may have a food sensitivity. You can move on to the challenge-testing phase, reintroducing foods one at a time. If a food produces a migraine attack, test it again. If you still react, you are probably intolerant to the food and need to cut it out.

If you don't react to a food, you can safely reintroduce it and move on to test the next food, and so on until all 'safe' foods have been reintroduced.

If you feel that you have identified all your personal food triggers and are feeling much better, there is no need to move on to a stricter regime. All you need to do is ensure that you are eating a balanced, healthy diet. In Chapter Six, we shall be looking at safe, healthy substitutes for some of the foods which you may have had to cut out of your diet.

Phase 2: the basic elimination diet

If you don't feel any benefit from being on the basic healthy diet, it could be that you are intolerant to some of the foods it contains, such as dairy products or wheat, both of which are common culprits. The next step is to move on to a relatively easy elimination diet. It is more difficult than the basic diet, but should not be too rigorous for a healthy, determined adult to follow. In addition to the list of foods you cut out when you were following the healthy-eating diet, the following foods are 'banned'.

Banned foods

• all cereals - wheat and bread, rye, barley, oats, corn [maize] and rice if eaten regularly. (Beware hidden ingredients! Note that wheat is present in pasta, couscous, semolina, biscuits, cakes, pastry, bread, and in many packaged foods as a thickener. Corn is found in sweetcorn, cornflakes, cornflour, corn syrup, popcorn, polenta.)

- beef, chicken
- dairy products (and foods containing milk solids)
- margarine
- eggs
- soya
- citrus fruits
- Marmite,Vegemite, Bovril, Oxo stock cubes
- mushrooms
- yeast (present in some vitamin supplements, especially B vitamins, overripe fruits, hydrolized protein and alcohol)
- peanuts
- processed meats
- smoked meats
- curries, spicy foods
- coffee, tea, chocolate, cola
- sugar and artificial sweeteners
- food additives
- alcohol
- vinegar and pickles
- aspirin and related drugs

Foods allowed on the diet

- lamb, turkey, pork (unless one of your triggers), duck, goose, rabbit
- fresh vegetables, including potatoes
- rice
- fresh fruit
- beans, lentils, chick peas
- nuts (unless you eat a lot of them)
- herb teas
- bottled mineral water
- pure vegetable oil

This diet can be modified slightly if you know that one of the foods is a personal trigger. For example, you can exclude pork, and substitute chicken if you feel it is not a problem for you. You may also be able to eat fish without any bad effects (but avoid smoked fish).

Avoid milk substitutes such as soya, goat or sheep's milk at this stage, as they can all cause problems. These can be tried later on, if you establish cow's milk as a trigger.

The exclusion phase of the basic elimination diet can be followed for two or three weeks. Try to vary your diet. For example, don't eat tons of potatoes to make up for the lack of wheat bread, as this could compound any sensitivity problems. Try other starchy foods, such as chestnuts, turnips or millet. You can use arrowroot if you need a thickener for gravies and sauces.

If you feel worse initially, then feel better, this is probably because you have eliminated a culprit food. Wait until the end of the three-week period, then challenge-test individual foods to isolate the problem ingredients.

If you still feel ill, you may be sensitive to one of the foods you are continuing to eat: perhaps something that you are now eating more of, to compensate for a food you have given up. You could try rotating the foods in the diet to see if it makes a difference. If not, move on to the most rigorous elimination diet.

Phase 3: the rigorous elimination diet

Most people will not need to proceed to the more rigorous elimination diets, as by this stage they will have identified enough of their culprit foods to achieve an improvement in their health.

The exact design of this elimination diet will depend upon your own individual lifestyle and diet, and any culprit foods which you have already identified. The basic rule is to devise an eating plan that relies on at least a dozen different foods, taken from the various nutritional groups to give variety and balance. This type of diet is sometimes called a 'rare foods diet' or 'few foods diet', as it is based on a small number of foods which you have either rarely eaten before, or have never eaten in any great quantity.

Below are some ideas for the sorts of food you might choose from. You will notice that they are not foods that most people consume in large amounts, but if they are foods that you particularly crave or dislike, you should not eat them on this diet.

- Meat and fish: rabbit, game, pheasant, venison, lamb, duck, goose, turkey.
- Vegetables: watercress, swede, alfalfa, okra, asparagus, spinach, fennel, celery, celeriac, lettuce.
- Fruit: any unusual fruits, excluding citrus – gooseberries, blackcurrants, redcurrants, kiwis, nashi pears, kiwano, lychees, mangoes, pomegranates, guavas, star fruit, passion fruit, rambutans, pears and so on.
- Starchy foods: millet, rice, buckwheat (no relation to wheat), turnips, parsnips, sweet potatoes, yams, wild rice, tapioca, sago, chestnuts, chickpeas, pumpkin.
- Fats and oils: olive, sunflower, safflower, rapeseed, coconut oil, creamed coconut.
- Snack foods: nuts (pistachios, brazils, cashews, pine nuts, macadamia - if you are not sensitive to them); pumpkin and sunflower seeds, unsulphured dried fruit.
- Drinks: bottled water and herb teas.

What to watch out for

If you feel initially worse, than better, you have probably eliminated one or more culprit foods. When you have been well for three or four days, you can begin challenge-testing.

If you don't derive any benefit from this diet, it is unlikely that you have a problem with food sensitivity. If you wish, you could try one of the more extreme elimination diets, such as the Stone Age Diet, the semi-fast the fast, or try a diet based only on foods that you have never eaten before. But never follow a fast or semi-fast for more than a few days at a time. If, at the end of this time, you still feel ill, consult your doctor.

Rescue remedy!

If you get a bad reaction to a food in a challenge test, you may find that a mixture of sodium bicarbonate (two teaspoonfuls) and potassium bicarbonate (one teaspoonful), dissolved in a glass of warm water, will help you to feel better more quickly. You can buy this mixture, under the trade name of Turnoff Allergy Treatment, from your health-food store or by mail order. Don't take this mixture too often, or after a heavy meal.

Elemental diets are formula diets, a little similar to baby formula, which have been developed for use by doctors with patients who have severe or multiple problems with food intolerance. Very much the last resort, they are not a substitute for a proper, balanced diet, and should not be tried except under full medical supervision.

Other types of elimination diet
These are variations on a theme, and should not be attempted for more than seven to fourteen days.

The eight-foods diet
On this you are allowed to choose from the following:

- turkey, rabbit
- spinach, turnip
- mango, kiwi
- buckwheat, millet
- sea salt
- bottled spring water.

The semi-fast
On this very monotonous diet you eat only two foods, for example lamb and pears, and drink only bottled spring water. Choose two foods that you are unlikely to be sensitive to, as you do not often eat them and do not particularly crave or dislike them.

The fruit
Some experts feel that the best way to begin an elimination diet is to fast for three to five days, taking only bottled spring water, with perhaps the addition of fresh fruit juices and/or herbal teas. The fasting process helps to get rid of toxins and allergens from the body quickly, particularly if the bowels are kept open.

However, fasting is inadvisable for migraine sufferers. Even people who do not suffer from migraine may find that they develop bad headaches during the first few days, and the low blood sugar levels are liable to provoke migraine attacks in those who are susceptible.

Fasting is probably best regarded as a last resort, when all other forms of exclusion diet have failed. In most cases, a semi-fast or rigorous elimination diet will be just as effective. Fasting is an extreme measure, and should not be undertaken for more than seven days at a time. Certain people should never fast:

- elderly people
- people whose general health is poor
- people who are underweight
- people with diabetes
- people suffering from epilepsy
- pregnant and nursing mothers
- children.

Always consult your GP if you are thinking of going on a fast, even for a couple of days, particularly if you are taking regular prescribed medication.

> NOTE: None of these elimination diets or fasts is designed to be followed for long periods. They are diagnostic aids, to help you identify and cut out any food triggers which may be contributing to your migraine. In the longer term, it is vital that you develop a good balanced diet that provides everything your body needs – and variety is important if you are to avoid developing further food sensitivities in months and years to come.

In Chapter Six, we shall be looking at varying your diet, at ways of creating a balanced and interesting diet, and finding healthy, tasty substitutes for your 'culprit' foods.

Know your food families

As many foods belong to 'families' of related animals and plants, there is always a chance of cross-sensitivity – that other foods from the same family may trigger migraine attacks. For example, if you are intolerant to potatoes, you could also be sensitive to tomatoes and aubergines that are closely related. If you are sensitive to chicken, you may also have a problem with eggs.

The list below contains some of the common members of different food families. It is worth checking to see if you are sensitive to more than one member of a family.

Wheat: wheat bran, flour, grains, semolina, bran, breakfast cereals. You could also be sensitive to other cereals such as, rye, barley, oats and corn.

- Gluten: wheat, barley, oats, rye, flour.
- Corn: corn (maize), sweetcorn, cornflour, corn syrup, popcorn, glucose syrup, corn oil, dextrose, baking powder, bottled sauces, baked beans, cornflakes, custard powder, margarine, polenta, tortillas.
- Yeast: brewer's and baker's yeast, beer, alcohol, over-ripe fruit, leavened bread, cheese, yoghurt, buttermilk, soured cream, yeast extract, stock cubes, beef extract, dried fruits, malt, malted drinks, vinegar, pickles, grapes, mouldy foods, mushrooms, fruit juices (except freshly squeezed).
- Colourings: tartrazine, fizzy and fruit drinks, pickles, bottled sauces, most processed and packaged foods, shop-bought cakes and mixes, soups, sauce mixes, custard powder, canned custard, instant puddings, sweets, filled chocolates, jelly, ice cream, ice lollies, jam, mustard.
- Preservatives: wines, chilled fruit juices, pickled onions, almost all processed foods, dried fruit, commercial pre-cut chips.
- Potatoes, potatoes, tomatoes, aubergines, peppers, chillies.
- Chicken: chicken, stock cubes, eggs, lecithin.
- Milk and beef: beef, suet, stock cubes, meat extracts, milk, milk chocolate, dairy foods, casein (milk protein), whey powder, milk solids, lactalbumen.
- Caffeine: coffee, tea, chocolate, cocoa, cola.

Environmental triggers

If you are feeling only partly better, or have not responded to the elimination diets, you may find it worthwhile to look around you for possible environmental triggers. These can be anything from cleaning products to perfumes, cigarette smoke to air pollution. One allergy expert claims that 'if you can smell it, it can do you harm'.

Obviously it's important not to become obsessive about triggers – food or otherwise – but it's certainly true that migraine sufferers can be sensitive to apparently innocuous substances in the everyday world around them. Sometimes this can take the form of allergy (to dust mite, airborne moulds or pollen), as often a subtler chemical sensitivity (developing a migraine after smelling wet gloss paint). Sometimes it is just a case of finding strong smells unbearable to the point of nausea, particularly in the hours leading up to an attack.

After years of unexplained migraines, my partner discovered one of his prime triggers to be Windolenea window cleaning liquid. With me, it tends to be petrol fumes, gloss paint and the perfume counter in department stores! Triggers vary widely from person to person, and some migraine sufferers are not at all sensitive to strong smells or chemicals.

Signs that suggest you may have a chemical sensitivity

- Certain smells make you feel good, give you a bit of a boost
- Strong smells, paint or perfume, give you a headache
- You were always car sick as a child, and even now get queasy on long journeys
- You keep feeling ill in the same place (at work).

Substances which may trigger migraine attacks in some sufferers

- aerosols
- household cleaners, detergents, disinfectants
- fuel
- gas leaks
- car interiors
- warm plastic
- cosmetics
- paints
- carpet and floor coverings
- foam rubber
- cavity wall insulation
- solvents (white spirit, methylated spirits)
- pet hair

- animal urine (especially mice, rats)
- household dust mite
- pollen
- airborne moulds.

Getting help from the experts

Your GP
It is very important to get support and practical help from your family doctor at the outset. Unfortunately, not all doctors are as sympathetic as they might be towards migraine sufferers in general and food intolerance problems in particular – so it's up to you to explain what you intend to do and ask for the help to which you are entitled.

After all, if your self-help programme works and you discover that you do have certain food intolerances or sensitivities, you have a very real chance of getting better without long-term prescription drugs. Most doctors welcome the chance to reduce their drugs bill!

Consult your doctor every step of the way, and don't be afraid to ask for additional help from a specialist or dietician if you need it, particularly in the post-diet stage when you are trying to devise a healthy eating plan. Point out to your doctor that, even if you end up discovering that you have no food intolerance problems, you will:

- feel better because you have done something to help yourself
- feel better because you have looked in detail at your diet and improved its nutritional value through healthier food choices
- feel better because you are freed from the fear that you will eat something which will bring on a migraine attack.

Specialists
Some doctors will be willing to offer additional help, in the form of a referral to an allergy specialist, although not all doctors will be keen. There are a few doctors who have a special interest in food allergy and intolerance, and in the relationship between food and migraine. Details of where to ask for information are given in the address section at the back of this book.

Clinical ecologists are people who specialize in treating allergy problems (and they often use the term 'allergy' to cover both allergy and intolerance). Some are qualified doctors, some are not. It is safest to ask for a referral from your doctor to be sure of getting informed and qualified help.

Total environmental control units
There are few total environmental control units in Britain, but there is a superb example in the Airedale Allergy Centre, near Bradford. The unit is run by an NHS consultant and accepts referrals from doctors on an NHS and private basis.

Here, they treat patients in a purpose-built clinic, most as outpatients but in severe cases on an in-patient basis as well. Every aspect of the patient's food and environment is controlled, and they have an impressive success rate with severe cases. In many instances they find that migraines are triggered by a combination of environmental and food sensitivities, so it is definitely worth studying all aspects of your lifestyle if a purely food-based approach doesn't work for you.

You must have a doctor's referral to attend the clinic, and not every doctor is eager to comply.

Allergy therapists
Allergy therapists come in all shapes and sizes. Some are qualified doctors, some qualified in alternative medicine, and others may not be qualified at all. The methods they use can be quite diverse. So finding the right therapist can be difficult.

One solution is to approach the Institute of Allergy Therapists, which keeps a register of around 150 members, most of them trained either in orthodox or complementary therapies. Members include doctors, osteopaths and reflexologists, but all are united in their approach to treating allergies and intolerances.

All members of the Institute use the same technique for the diagnosis and treatment of allergies and intolerance. First of all, the patient's intolerances are identified; these are then treated using a form of homeopathic desensitization. The remedies used are made in the Institute's own homeopathic pharmacy.

When this stage is complete, the therapist takes a close look at the migraine sufferer's lifestyle and suggestions are made for reducing stress, as this is regarded as an important element in provoking migraine attacks.

The Institute can refer members of the public to an allergy therapist in their area, and address details are given at the end of this book.

Treatments for food intolerance

As we have seen, simply eliminating the foods that make you ill can be a very successful way of dealing with your food intolerance problems – and so helping your migraine. However, this can be a little boring and restrictive, and some doctors and other specialists offer treatments which could make it possible to eat culprit foods without the serious side effect of a migraine attack. These treatments are mainly of value in cases of food allergy, but may have some value in the treatment of food intolerance.

Desensitization

In the past, this treatment was frequently offered to allergy sufferers by their GPs. The principle is that progressively stronger injections of the substance that produces an allergy will eventually desensitize the patient to that substance.

The treatment is no longer offered by GPs, as it has been proved to be dangerous – in fact, fatal – in some cases. In most cases it simply doesn't work, and there is no reason to think that it would be much of use in cases of food intolerance (as opposed to allergy).

Provocation and neutralization

This is also known as serial end-point skin titration, or Miller's Method, and it has been developed from the skin-prick allergy test.

A dilution of a suspect substance is injected into the skin, producing a weal. If it grows, compared to a control weal, then this suggests there is an allergy. The reaction is treated by injecting progressively weaker dilutions of the substance into the skin, until the weal stops growing and any symptoms disappear. This dosage is called the 'switch-off' or neutralizing dose, and it acts as a sort of antidote to the substance.

Patients can be given a cocktail of the diluted substance, which they either inject or put under the tongue, before they eat the problem foods. It is a much safer method than desensitization because the injections are progressively weaker.

Sublingual provocation and neutralization

This is similar to provocation and neutralization, but drops are put under the tongue instead of the substance being injected. It is useful for children who are afraid of injections.

Enzyme potentiated desensitization

In enzyme potentiated desensitization (EPD), the forearm is scratched to remove the surface layer of skin. A cup containing a cocktail of diluted allergens is taped over the skin and left in place for 24 hours.

The substances soak into the blood and antibodies are produced. Practitioners claim an 85 per cent success rate with allergy sufferers, over a period of months.

Coming to terms with food intolerance

Once you have identified the problem foods that are contributing to your migraine attacks, you need to develop a strategy which will give you a healthy, migraine-free future. In most cases, this will mean modifying your diet on a long-term basis. In Chapter Six, we shall be looking at ways of changing the way you eat, and developing an enjoyable, nutritious diet that will not leave you feeling deprived or restricted.

Chapter Five

Migraine? No problem!

By this stage, you will know whether or not your migraine is associated with eating certain foods. The natural next step is to cut those foods out of your diet, but sometimes this can cause problems in itself. Even following a basic, healthy diet can be problematic if the rest of the family wants to go to McDonald's. In this chapter, we take a look at these problems and suggest some ways in which they can be overcome.

This chapter is intended to be used as a resource. There are no absolutes, and you will need to find your own solutions. But I do hope that you will find some useful tips for a migraine-free lifestyle.

Cravings

A little of what you fancy may do you good, but unfortunately it's not necessarily true if you suffer from migraine.

Many migraine sufferers endure the most horrendous cravings – often for the very foods that trigger their attacks. It can be really frustrating, having to deny yourself your favourite 'comfort' foods, because you strongly suspect that they will make you ill.

The good news is that it may not always be necessary to deny yourself all of your problem foods. Quite a few female sufferers find that they can eat foods like chocolate without problems, except in the days leading up to a period, when they are particularly susceptible to migraine attacks. Personally, I find that I can eat small amounts of very mild, unmatured cheese without problems, except in the week before my menstrual period, when I seem to be particularly sensitive to dairy products and fatty foods.

Others can eat trigger foods except at times of exceptional stress, or find that they are unaffected unless they eat large amounts of the food on an empty stomach.

Some people find that cravings are a sort of warning sign that they are in danger of having an attack. Their food cravings occur only at times when it would be a very bad idea to eat the food. This is a particularly nasty irony of nature, but at least this way you can learn to pinpoint the times when you really mustn't give in to the urge to scoff an entire box of chocolates, or half a pound of mature cheddar.

Remember that it generally takes more than one trigger to start a migraine attack. For example, cheese plus stress plus menstrual period may well result in an attack, whereas cheese on its own, with no other precipitating factors, may cause no problems at all.

As time goes on, you will learn how far you can go in satisfying your desire for certain foods. Here are the general rules.

- Beware of giving in to very strong cravings: they could be a warning sign that you are vulnerable to an attack.
- Find out, by trial and error, whether you are sensitive to your problem foods all the time, or only at certain specific times or in identifiable situations.
- If you find that you can eat the food safely at certain times, indulge yourself ... in moderation.
- Don't go mad and eat large amounts of any food: even if you get away with it on one occasion, you risk a bad reaction the next time you eat the food.
- Even foods to which you are not sensitive should not be eaten every day: you risk developing an intolerance.

Dining in style

Informal entertaining
Entertaining, or visiting friends for a meal, can pose a few problems for the migraine sufferer.

It can be excruciatingly embarrassing having to ask for special treatment, particularly if you're visiting someone you don't know very well, but the best thing really is to explain at the outset. It's much better to give a clear explanation of the things you can't eat when you receive the invitation, rather than to wait for the night and then have to refuse all the carefully prepared dishes – or, worse, eat them and then suffer a migraine attack later.

Most people are very happy to accommodate your needs, and if you are eating with close friends you could even offer to take along your own food. Often, all that needs to be done is to offer an alternative vegetable or fruit, or to serve any sauces separately so that you can choose whether or not to indulge.

Don't be afraid to tell people about your needs, and don't be persuaded that 'it'll be all right just this once'. If a food makes you ill, you shouldn't eat it just to be polite. Be firm, assertive, give a clear explanation, and everything will be fine.

Official functions

On occasion, you may need to attend an official dinner or function where you will have no choice over the food available. This can certainly be difficult, but if you are selective about what you eat, you should be OK. Avoid sauces and opt for plain meats and boiled or steamed vegetables. Fruit may be your best option for dessert. Watch out for vegetarian alternatives, as they are often packed full of cheese.

Just in case the worst happens, and you find you really can't risk eating anything, be prepared! Missing meals is a very bad idea for migraine sufferers, so you need to plan ways of preventing hypoglycaemia.

Before eating out (particularly if you're going to be eating late), always have a light, starchy snack. A few dry crackers or a small portion of plain boiled rice or pasta is perfect, but anything will do as long as it is not a sugary or salty processed product.

This way, you will raise your blood sugar level and you will be able to last longer if you can't eat the set meal.

If you take another small snack along with you, you can sneak into the cloakroom and eat it, should you find you have to go without your dinner. Again, a starchy snack, perhaps a fruit bar or even a tub of cottage cheese is ideal – something portable and easily digested. You can then dance the night away and not worry!

Restaurants

Obviously it may not be possible to view the menu before you go to the restaurant, but you should be able to choose a type of restaurant which will accommodate your personal needs.

If you are sensitive to spicy foods, garlic or chillies you will probably wish to avoid Indian, Thai or Mexican food.

Chinese food can, of course, be problematic because of the high levels of monosodium glutamate. Crispy duck may be OK, but if you are very sensitive to MSG you may wish to give Chinese food a miss. Some people are only affected by MSG if they consume it on an empty stomach. Eating a snack before you go will help to raise blood sugar levels, and you may find filling up on plain boiled rice damps down any reaction.

Cheese is a common element in many Italian, Mexican and American foods – and is often a hidden ingredient. Hidden ingredients can crop up in the most unexpected places, particularly as many restaurant dishes are not cooked on the premises but pre prepared in a factory then reheated on site.

Don't be afraid to ask the waiter about any ingredients in the dishes. If he can't answer – or if you suspect he doesn't really know but isn't saying – opt for something really plain and simple, with ingredients you know won't pose problems for you. Alternatively, ask for a dish to be modified (e.g. without the grilled cheese topping), and stress that if your instructions are not followed to the letter, you will be very ill. Most restaurants will not take a chance and cheat, because they are afraid you will collapse in their restaurant, or sue them for thousands of pounds in compensation!

I love pizza, but can't risk too much cheese. Asking for pizza without cheese does produce a few raised eyebrows, but you soon get used to doing it – and, as far as I'm concerned, it's a great deal better than doing without pizza altogether! Incidentally, mozzarella is a very mild cheese and you may find you have no problems with it. Unfortunately, quite a few restaurants mix Cheddar with the mozzarella because it is cheaper and stronger tasting. If in doubt, do without the cheese altogether.

Of course, restaurants aren't always co-operative. I once asked for a homemade burger without cheese in quite a smart restaurant. In due course it arrived – smothered in melted cheese. I pointed out that this wasn't what I'd ordered, and that cheese makes me ill, and the waitress took it away, promising to replace it. Five minutes later it reappeared: not a freshly cooked burger, but the old one with the cheese half-scraped off! You could still see stringy bits of melted cheese hanging off the burger!

The temptation was, of course, to eat the burger – especially as the other people at my table were halfway through their meal by now – but I didn't dare. So I complained and in the end I did get a new burger. But I didn't visit that restaurant again!

This story serves to illustrate that a lot of people still don't have a clue about migraine – how it works, or what it feels like. They think that when we ask for something without cheese, we're just being fussy. It's our job to re-educate them, not to keep quiet and suffer in silence.

The foods that you choose from a restaurant menu will, of course, vary according to your personal migraine triggers, but I find that omelettes, pure beefburgers, salads (watch out for the citrus fruits), grilled fish and grilled and roast meats are usually OK for me. However, garlic is a real disaster for me although for some inexplicable reason it has no effect on me if I eat it in Indian food. I am very careful to avoid garlic-laden marinades, which may also contain soy sauce, a trigger for some people who have problems with MSG. If you are sensitive to wheat, be careful with thick sauces and soups. The basic rule is: don't eat too much of anything, and don't risk eating something if you don't know what's in it.

Fast food

If you're lucky, the odd visit to McDonald's won't do you too much damage. Some of the fast-food chains publish leaflets giving nutritional details about the foods they sell, so you may be able to check up on additives and other ingredients in advance. Burger King make a point of saying that customers can have their burgers any way they want them, with any combination of ingredients – definitely a challenge worth taking up!

Some forms of fast food, such as baked potatoes, are unlikely to do you any harm, but watch out for additive-laden fillings. I once had a nasty migraine attack after eating a jacket potato filled with 'home-made' chilli con carne that was actually out of a tin. The same applies to French-style crepes, although these need to be avoided it you are sensitive to wheat.

Burgers and hot dogs sold from roadside vans are almost certainly a bad idea, and I would avoid them like the plague. Cheap ingredients and lots of additives make for a migraine sufferer's nightmare.

Shopping

Before you next go shopping, invest a little time in becoming the world's greatest expert at reading labels.

Packets and tins are a lot more informative about ingredients than they used to be, and if you spend a little extra time initially in getting to know different products, you will soon get the hang of what you can and can't eat. A book like E for Additives may help you find your way around the labels.

Unfortunately, manufacturers often use scientific jargon and techno-speak when they are compiling food labels, so a fairly ordinary ingredient can be listed under a variety of quite exotic names. Ingredients derived from milk, for example, might appear as milk solids, whey solids, lactalbumen or casein.

Below is a list of some common foods, together with some of the technical names that may indicate their presence in a food:

Wheat
- cereal protein
- food starch
- flour
- cereal binder
- cereal starch
- edible starch
- modified starch
- baking powder

Corn (maize)
- modified starch
- corn starch
- corn meal
- vegetable gum
- food starch
- cereal starch
- corn syrup
- dextrose
- edible starch
- glucose syrup
- vegetable oil
- baking powder

Milk
- casein
- caseinate
- whey
- lactalbumen
- lactose

Egg
- ovalbumen
- lecithin

Yeast
- leavening
- raising agent (may be baking powder)
- hydroliyzed [vegetable] protein

Sugar
- dextrose
- lactose
- frutose
- glucose
- maltose
- sucrose

Soya
- textured vegetable protein (TVP)
- tofu
- vegetable protein
- [soya] lecithin
- miso
- vegetable gum

Drinking

Drinking isn't just about consuming alcohol: it's about socializing and being one of the gang. If you don't have a glass in your hand at a party, or by your plate at the dinner table, it's easy to feel like the odd one out.

Few people have to avoid alcohol completely, but avoid red wine (particularly cheap varieties), and drink all forms of alcohol sparingly. One good tip is to have a glass of mineral water and glass of wine going at the same time. You can take little sips of wine, punctuated by larger gulps of water, which will help to dilute the volume of alcohol you consume. Another option is to follow the French custom of diluting your wine with an equal volume of water.

There are also a good many more credible alcohol substitutes than there used to be, including de-alcoholized wines. Perhaps a better (and more palatable) option is red or white grape juice, which is very wine-like in appearance. Low-alcohol beers may still cause problems for some migraine sufferers, because they contain various substances beside alcohol (malt, yeast).

One of my favourite non-alcoholic drinks is elderflower

'champagne', or elderflower pressé. You can make your own, using fresh elderflowers and lemons, or buy it in health-food shops, delicatessens and supermarkets. An economical alternative is to buy concentrated elderflower cordial and dilute it with still or sparkling mineral water. The resulting drink looks and tastes quite similar to white wine, and is delicious served very cold. I find it soothing and refreshing, even when I have an attack coming on and can't tolerate tea or coffee.

Exercise

Many migraine sufferers find that strenuous or prolonged exercise lowers their blood sugar level and makes them more prone to attacks.

Try taking a glucose tablet (or teaspoon of glucose) before exercising, and a starchy snack within half an hour of finishing. This should help to compensate for lost energy.

Finding 'safe' substitutes

Obviously it isn't a good idea to cut valuable foods out of your diet without finding suitably nutritious substitutes. To subsist on a restricted diet over a long period isn't just dangerous in terms of essential nutrients. It's also putting you at risk of developing further food sensitivities – and what's the point of swapping one set of sensitivities for another?

Then there are the potential psychological effects of denying yourself a varied and interesting diet. Some migraine sufferers have become so anxious and obsessive because of the fear of making themselves ill that they have reduced their diet to ridiculous and dangerous levels. One allergist reported that a patient was subsisting on nothing but tea, toast and lettuce: clearly a bad idea, no matter what the circumstances.

As soon as you have determined which foods are your triggers, you must set about finding new foods, which you can add to your diet, to take their place. The more varied your diet, the less frequently you will eat each individual food, and the less risk you will run of developing any further food problems.

If you wish, you can ask a nutritionist or dietician to help you devise a rotation diet, in which members of the same food families are only eaten at four- or five-day intervals. Experts use this rotation system to help prevent new food sensitivities developing.

How easy it is to find substitutes depends very much upon the foods you have to give up. We might not want to live without chocolate, but nutritionally speaking it's hardly an essential element of anyone's diet. On the other hand, giving up wheat can be a bigger problem, particularly if you find you are sensitive to other cereals or other types of cereal gluten. Giving up bread, crackers, sauces, breakfast cereal and a whole host of other wheat-related products can mean making some pretty substantial changes to your diet. But it can be done! And what's more, it can be done without condemning yourself to a boring or unduly restrictive diet. You may also discover that you develop a taste for new and exotic flavours. The keynote is experimentation.

In the Further Reading section of this book, you will find a list of 'alternative' cookery books, which contain recipes suitable for migraine sufferers with a variety of different food problems. Select some of these recipes and try them out. Learn to produce tasty, nutritious food using new ingredients, and once you have established a repertoire of menus, you will find that you can even throw a swish dinner party without anyone realizing they're eating 'special' food. And that is exactly how it should be. The aim is not to be different from other people, but to be happy, integrated, well nourished and free from anxieties which might develop into obsessions.

Discussed below are of some of the foods, which may cause problems for some migraine sufferers, together with suggested substitutes. Some you will find in ordinary supermarkets, some in health-food stores, and others are available by mail order.

Chocolate and sweets

Nobody actually needs to eat chocolate, so if this is the only thing you need to cut down on, consider yourself lucky! Nevertheless, most of us derive a lot of comfort from eating chocolate, and it can be quite a wrench to give it up.

The most commonly advocated substitute is carob, a type of naturally sweet, ground-up beanpod. This may not sound very appetizing, but in fact it is fairly palatable and can be made into bars which have a very similar consistency to chocolate. There are dairy-free carob bars, no-added-sugar carob bars, carob drops and even filled non-dairy 'chocolates' for those who are sensitive to milk. You can buy carob powder, which is rather like fine cocoa powder in consistency, and gives good results in baking.

If you have milk intolerance, but are OK with soya, you might like to try Granymels, which are a sort of dairy-free toffee, available in a variety of flavours from health-food stores or by mail order.

If milk is not your problem, there are plenty of things to try: fudge, toffee, boiled sweets, coconut ice – the list is endless. Some migraineurs find liquorice a problem, so you may wish to avoid it. If you cannot eat a lot of sugar, sugar-free sweets and no-added-sugar carob bars may be the answer. Boots now sell a range of 'tooth-friendly', sugar-free confectionery approved by the British Dental Association.

Avoid eating a lot of sweets containing the artificial sweetener sorbitol, as this can have a laxative effect.

Drinks containing caffeine

Tea, coffee, chocolate, cocoa and cola drinks all contain significant amounts of caffeine. 'Real' coffee is the worst offender (with around 85mg per cupful), while hot chocolate contains only around 4mg for an equivalent cupful. Cola drinks vary, with 'own brands' generally lower in caffeine than Coca-Cola or Pepsi – although this may change with the introduction of supermarket 'traditional' colas. Brands of caffeine-free and sugar-free cola are now available if you want to give up but miss the taste too much, but watch out for legions of additives.

Decaffeinated tea and coffee are both available, and taste much better than they used to. However, some people may find that other substances in tea and coffee, besides the caffeine, can cause headaches. Why not try one of the alternative instant drinks on sale in health-food shops? Dandelion coffee, Bambu, Caro, Barleycup and herbal teas are all worth a try, and will help you to reduce your caffeine level. Rooibosch (Redbush) Tea or Mate Tea are useful alternatives to 'real' tea.

Cheese

This is one of the hardest foods to substitute, as it has such a unique taste and texture, and is both very nutritious and convenient to use.

If you really can't live without cheese, keep to low-tyramine or non-tyramine types, such as cottage, quark, Philadelphia, cream and curd. You can also experiment with sheep's and goat's cheeses, some of which are very fresh and mild. Mild cheeses like Wensleydale and Cheshire may be tolerated in small amounts, but steer clear of powerful, matured cheeses and blue cheeses like Stilton and Gorgonzola. The riper (and smellier) a cheese is, the more likely it is to cause you problems.

I find Dairylea cheese spread is OK in moderation. You can make a passable Welsh rarebit using mainly curd or cottage cheese, plus a little grated hard cheese.

Gjetost is a rather peculiar Norwegian brown cheese, made from milk whey. It contains no casein, and may be tolerated even if you have a milk or cheese sensitivity. The only drawback is that it doesn't taste much like cheese!

Sunflower and soya cheeses are both available in health-food stores. Sunflower cheese may still cause problems in some people, but it tastes quite nice, if a little rubbery (a bit like Havarti). The kindest thing I can say about soya cheese is that it is an acquired taste which I have not yet managed to acquire. It certainly doesn't taste much like cheese. There are also soya 'yoghurts' and 'cheese spreads'. Another soya product is tofu, which can be bought marinated and/or smoked, but be careful if you are sensitive to smoked foods or to ingredients in the marinade. You can buy plain tofu and flavour it with your own marinade.

Possibly a tastier alternative are savoury spreads. If you are not sensitive to yeast, you could try Vessen or Tartex vegetarian paté, available from health-food stores. There are also tofu-based spreads. Meat-based spreads and patés could pose problems because of additives and their pork/bacon content. Other options include peanut and other 'butters': sunflower, cashew, hazelnut, and tahini (made from sesame seeds).

Cooked turkey makes a good alternative to cheese or ham in sandwiches, but all shop-bought cooked meats are liable to contain added nitrates and water.

Milk

If you have an intolerance to cow's milk, it is worth trying evaporated milk, which some people can tolerate. Goat's milk can be tried, although this too can cause problems. Sheep's milk has a pleasanter, creamier taste and may be less prone to provoke allergy and intolerance problems. Soya milk is another option, but check for soya intolerance first. Soya milk can be made at home, using soya flour.

As an alternative to butter, there are plenty of poly- and monounsaturated margarines and spreads, but watch out for those containing whey/milk solids (e.g. Flora). Some people like to follow the Mediterranean custom of moistening bread with olive oil. If you put olive oil into the refrigerator it will solidify and you can use it as a spread.

Wheat
Some people are intolerant to gluten, which is also present in rye, barley and oats, so if you have a problem with wheat, you'll need to test these, too.

There are other alternatives to wheat, many of which can be milled into flour for use in baking. The only real problem is that it is the gluten in wheat which makes it sticky and therefore good for baking. Flours which do not contain gluten tend to crumble and don't bind together well, so you will either have to use a proportion of another 'sticky' flour (such as gram or soya) or bind with egg or an egg substitute such as Bipro.

It is well worth trying rye, barley, rice or millet flours. And you can also try non-cereal flours such as buckwheat (no relation to wheat), soya, pea, quinoa, sago, potato, chickpea or chestnut. These may not be tremendously successful if used on their own in baking, but in combinations they can be quite satisfactory. If you can tolerate corn (maize), a proportion of cornflour will help to lighten your baking. A number of wheat-free cookery books are available.

If you don't fancy baking, you can make grain porridge and eat it with fruit or savoury foods (maize and millet work quite well). Alternatively, your health-food store or chemist may be able to supply proprietary wheat-free breads, cakes, baking mixes and biscuits.

If you buy rye bread, make sure that it contains only rye; many shop-bought loaves contain some wheat flour. Alternatives to bread include rice cakes (which taste a bit like Sugar Puffs without the sugar), pure rye crispbreads and oatcakes. You can now buy pasta and/or noodles made from rice, buckwheat and other flours.

Baking powder may contain wheat or corn flour. You can make your own by mixing two ounces of bicarbonate of soda with four and a half ounces of cream of tartar, plus two ounces of another flour (rice, for example).

Yeast
Try unleavened bread and crackers. Some pitta breads contain yeast – check the packet for ingredients. You could also try making your own soda bread. Health-food shops now sell yeast-free vegetable bouillon cubes for stews, gravies, sauces and casseroles.

Alcohol
Avoid all red wine, with the possible exception of good vintage reds, which may turn out to be problem-free. Try grape juice or elderflower drinks. Drink lots of water, and consider diluting your wine to reduce your intake. 'Pure' spirits such as vodka or gin may be tolerated.

Citrus fruit
Try other fruits rich in vitamin C, such as kiwis, melons, and blackcurrants, which can give good, strong flavours. Raspberries are good if you are not sensitive to them. Good-quality malt or cider vinegar can replace lemon juice in baking.

Eggs
There are a variety of egg-replacement products on the market, including Bipro, which is made from milk. Alternatively, you could try using gelatine in cooking.

Coping during a migraine attack

Now and then, we all experience those familiar warning signs which tell us another migraine attack is on the way. But even at this pre-attack stage it is possible to use food and drink to help minimize the pain and disruption of an attack. Here are some tips to help you weather the storm.

- Find a drink which you can tolerate and drink as much fluid as you can as soon as you know you are about to have an attack. Plain water is fine, but some people prefer tea, or fizzy drinks like lemonade or Lucozade. The caffeine in tea and strong coffee may help by giving a temporary 'lift'.

- Fizzy drinks may help: you can dissolve soluble pain-relievers in a glass of lemonade and the fizziness seems to aid absorption of the painkiller. Remember to take your medication early on in the attack, for maximum effect.
- Try eating a plain, cooked meal as soon as you get the first warning signs. This is sometimes enough to abort an attack. Go for simple foods and avoid fat.
- If your doctor has given you drugs to improve gastric motility, take them early on in the attack.
- Some people find that kelp tablets are helpful.
- Glucose tablets may give a much needed emergency boost to a critically low blood sugar level. But don't take sugar routinely, or you will tend to make your blood sugar problems worse.
- Herbal teas, infusions and tisanes may be soothing. In the next chapter we shall discuss these in more detail.

Chapter Six

A menu for living

Even if you've discovered that you don't suffer from specific food sensitivities, avoiding foods which are known to contain headache-producing substances may reduce your chances of having an attack. Eating regularly, and eating the right things, can also protect you against getting ill. What's more, your overall health will certainly benefit from a more nutritious, balanced diet and gentle exercise, and a healthier lifestyle can make difference to the way you feel.

The message of this book is that prevention is better than cure; and there is a lot you can do, through diet, exercise and life-style management, to protect yourself from the pain and disruption of attacks. Why not give it a try? You have absolutely nothing to lose, and everything to gain.

Migraine and your health

Many experts have concluded that improving your general health is an excellent way of combating migraine. This doesn't mean rigorous dieting or strenuous exercise; it means taking a long, hard look at your diet, fitness and lifestyle, and making adjustments that will make you feel better without too much hardship on your part. The key is moderation in all things. If you aren't happy with what you're doing, then don't do it. Your unhappiness will only be an additional source of unwanted stress . . . and we all know what stress can do to us as migraine sufferers.

Adopting a healthier lifestyle can have a number of beneficial effects for migraine sufferers – and their families!

Diet

- A diet rich in vitamins, minerals and essential fatty acids should correct any nutritional deficiencies which are contributing to your illness, and build up your resistance. If you are following any sort of restricted diet, you will need to be careful to ensure that you are getting all the nutrients your body needs.

- Dietary fibre, from fresh fruit and vegetables, cereals etc will help to promote a healthy gut and speedily eliminate any toxins or problem foods from the body.
- Eating plenty of unrefined carbohydrates, and avoiding large amounts of sugar, should help to correct any problems with low blood sugar. This in turn may help with premenstrual and menopausal symptoms.
- Cutting out junk foods and caffeine may help to reduce anxiety, a powerful migraine trigger.
- Avoiding fatty foods and foods containing known headache triggers (e.g. nitrates, MSG, caffeine, vaso-active amines) may reduce your susceptibility to attacks at times of stress and so on.
- Thinking about what you eat, and planning ahead, will help you to introduce variety into your diet. Experts say that eating a varied diet is essential for good health, and helps to reduce the risk of developing food intolerances.
- Whether you are under- or overweight, modifying your diet to make it more nutritious could help you to reach and sustain your ideal weight more easily. Better nutrition may help you to lose weight, as healthier foods tend to be more filling and sustaining.
- There is some evidence that eating carbohydrates rich in tryptophan may help to enhance the effect of the body's own endorphins, reducing pain – although in some cases, these tryptophan-rich foods can actually be a trigger for migraine attacks.

Dietary supplements

- Most people don't need to take supplements, and ideally you should be getting all your essential nutrients from the foods you eat. But supplements can be helpful if you have had to cut out an important food source (e.g. calcium supplements to replace dairy products).
- Certain supplements can be taken to help build up resistance and in some cases may help prevent attacks or reduce their severity.

Certain vitamins and minerals have proved particularly helpful.

- Herbal preparations can also be taken to ward off attacks, or to soothe and treat symptoms during an attack. The most famous of these is feverfew, but there are many other options worth trying.

Exercise and relaxation

- Gentle exercise will strengthen your muscles and improve circulation and general health.
- Exercises for the back, shoulders, neck and facial muscles may reduce muscle tension and headache. Stronger, more elastic muscles are much less likely to go into spasm.
- The Alexander Technique can improve posture and related headaches.
- Regular exercise helps the body to produce its own pain-relieving substances, called endorphins. These also promote a sense of wellbeing and reduce stress and anxiety.
- Learning relaxation, meditation, yoga or self-hypnosis can also reduce stress levels, removing an important migraine trigger.

Psychological benefits

- Taking better care of yourself helps to promote a much greater sense of self-esteem and self-worth.
- Eating regularly and healthily helps to even out mood swings.
- Cutting out trigger foods to which you are intolerant may also eliminate other symptoms (such as a runny nose, stomach ache and aching muscles), improving your overall sense of wellbeing.
- Cutting out caffeine will help to reduce anxiety and stress.
- Above all, you will feel that you are at last in control of your own body and your own health, instead of being at the mercy of your migraine.

Diet

Elimination diets are a useful way of finding out if you have food-related problems, but they are not designed to be followed for more than a few weeks at a time. Cutting out your trigger foods over a longer period of time could cause problems if those foods have a high nutritional value, so you must plan ahead and make sure that your body is getting everything it needs to function properly. If you take something of value out of your diet, then you must replace it with something of equal value.

For example, let's say you have discovered that cow's milk is a trigger. That may mean you have to eliminate not just milk but everything that has milk or milk solids in it: cheese, butter, yoghurt, casein, lactose – a whole host of nutritionally-valuable foods. Milk provides protein, calcium, vitamins and minerals; and you will certainly have to think about replacing lost calcium, either by eating lots of green vegetables or by taking a calcium supplement. Calcium deficiency in children and women can cause very serious bone problems.

What are the elements of a good, healthy diet?

In Chapter Four, we used a basic healthy diet as the first stage in eliminating possible problem foods. Most of us will not have to follow anything quite as strict in our ordinary daily lives. Doctors have put forward the following recommendations, which are simple to follow and which can be adapted to take account of your personal triggers.

- Foods you should eat often: fruit and vegetables: starches (bread, potatoes, grains, pasta, rice and so on).
- Foods you should eat in moderation: dairy products, meat, poultry, eggs, beans, nuts.
- Foods you should eat occasionally: fats, oils, sugars.

This simple healthy diet should offer a good balance of fats, proteins and carbohydrates, essential vitamins and minerals, as long as you vary the different foods you eat. A little of everything, in moderation: that's the golden rule. As a migraine sufferer, you may well wish to adapt the diet to eliminate such foods as cheese or citrus fruits, but be sure to replace these with other foods of equal nutritional value.

If in doubt, consult your doctor and ask to be referred to a dietician/ nutritionist. Don't take chances with your health.

General rules for healthier eating

- Cut down on salt, sugar, alcohol, fat, processed foods, caffeine and any personal food triggers.
- Eat more fibre, fresh fruit and vegetables.
- Don't overcook foods, or cook at unnecessarily high temperatures, as this can destroy vitamins. Add vegetables to boiling water – never put them into cold water and then heat up. Vegetable water may contain water-soluble vitamins, so use it in your cooking or drink it. Steaming vegetables keeps them firm and crisp, and helps preserve more of the vitamins.
- Eat some raw fruit and vegetables every day.
- Don't deep fry. You can dry-fry in a non-stick pan, or use a very small amount of oil.
- Grill or bake meat (e.g. in a terracotta pot), and cut off excess fat or poultry skin.
- Add taste to your recipes with herbs and spices.

Hypoglycaemia

Fluctuating blood sugar levels are a major trigger in migraine attacks, but these are effectively controlled by healthy eating. This strategy has been found to be particularly effective in preventing menstrually-related migraine attacks, and in treating women suffering from pre-menstrual syndrome (PMS). Here are the rules to follow.

- Eat little and often. Small, frequent meals are much better for everyone (not just hypoglycaemia sufferers), and offer a sustained source of energy throughout the day.
- Eat small, starchy snacks: but not sugary or processed foods. Crackers, rice, bread and pasta and all good, as are fruit, no-added-sugar cereal bars, potatoes, nuts and sunflower seeds. Avoid sugars and processed carbohydrates, as these will only make the problem worse.
- Fresh foods containing lots of natural fibre (e.g. fruit, vegetables, oats) will also help to even out your blood sugar levels. The type of dietary fibre found in oats is thought to play a part in protecting us against heart disease, as well as some types of bowel cancer.
- Never go for more than four or five hours without eating,

preferably no more than three hours. This is particularly important in the days leading up to a menstrual period.

- If you like to 'lie in' at the weekend, but find you wake with the beginnings of a migraine attack, set your alarm for your weekday time and keep a snack by the bed. When you wake eat the snack – you can then turn over and have a snooze!

- This applies to long, romantic sessions of lovemaking, too: if you're going to be spending hours in bed, using up lots of energy, you'll be at risk of an attack. Take some food to bed with you . . . and let your imagination run riot!

Caffeine

It makes sense to cut down on caffeine as far as possible, as it is a stimulant and can exacerbate stress and anxiety, compounding the effects of blood sugar problems.

Some experts suggest limiting your intake to around 600mg per day, some to as little as 200mg. When you consider that 'real' coffee contains around 85mg per cup, and tea around 40mg, it's easy to see that the enthusiastic tea, coffee or cola drinker could get through the day's ration in no time. Try caffeine-free drinks, as suggested in the previous chapter.

Some sufferers find that a caffeine boost helps them if they have the first signs of an attack, and some pain-relievers contain caffeine for this very reason.

Additives

Even if you don't have a problem with individual additives, it's worth avoiding them if you can – if only because we don't yet know the long-term effects of some commonly used substances. Try incorporating some organic foods into your diet. Or why not grow your own?

Dietary fibre

We all need to eat more fibre – but don't eat too much wheat bran, as this can hinder the absorption of calcium. Eat lots of wholemeal bread, fruit and vegetables and wholegrains. Oats are especially valuable as a rich source of soluble fibre.

A healthy gut will also help your body to rid itself quickly of any problem substances, and may guard against some bowel disorders.

Dietary supplements and herbal remedies

Health-food stores are packed to the ceilings with vitamin and mineral supplements, pills, potions and herbal remedies. But do we need them? Can they really do anything to help the migraine sufferer, or are they just part of a plot to make us part with our hard-earned cash?

The answer is that if you are in good health and eat a varied diet, you probably don't need dietary supplements for nutritional reasons. Doctors say that the only people who may need to take regular vitamin and mineral supplements are the elderly, children and pregnant and nursing women.

However, there is some evidence that taking selected vitamins and minerals can help to prevent migraine attacks. Also, daily requirements can and do vary between individuals and in different circumstances, and the Recommended Daily Amounts (RDAs) of vitamins tend to be the amounts necessary to prevent serious illnesses like scurvy, rather than the amount which will promote the best state of health. You may find that you need additional vitamins and/or minerals at times of stress, or in the days leading up to a menstrual period.

NOTE: If you have problems with food intolerance, you may need to steer clear of products that contain flavourings, colourings and the like. Many B vitamins are synthesized from yeast, and vitamin C products often contain citrus flavourings and colourings. Vitamin C is usually manufactured from corn, whilst vitamin E is derived from wheatgerm. Some health-food stores now stock hypo-allergenic supplements, which are less likely to cause a bad reaction. It is also possible to obtain yeast-free B-vitamins.

It is not advisable to take enormous amounts of vitamins A, D or B6, as in rare cases this could be harmful.

Supplements which some migraine sufferers have found helpful
Vitamins
Vitamins are essential to health, but can't be manufactured in our own bodies. They are often destroyed by over-cooking or by storing foods too long before eating them. (This is one of the major concerns

in the controversy over irradiated foods.)

The vitamins which have been found, by migraine sufferers, to be most useful are vitamins C, A, E, folic acid, pantothenic acid and vitamins B1, B6 and B12. Niacin has a vasodilatory effect and has been found to be useful in treating some cases of migraine, although in large doses it could trigger an attack.

Minerals

Some minerals are also essential to health, although we need only take in very small amounts to remain healthy.

The minerals which have been found by migraine sufferers to be most useful are: magnesium, chromium, selenium, zinc, iron and calcium. Magnesium may be useful in promoting muscle relaxation.

Essential fatty acids

These, too, cannot be manufactured in the body. The most famous source of EFAs is evening primrose oil, which contains linolenic acid. Some people have found it works well in relieving the symptoms of PMS and menstrually-related migraines. It works best if you are getting enough magnesium, vitamin C, zinc. Vitamin B6 and niacin.

Other sources of linolenic acid include safflower and sunflower oil.

Fish oil

In clinical trials at the University of Cincinnati, daily fish oil capsules were found to reduce the incidence of bad headaches by more than 50 per cent. An alternative is to eat lots of oily (but not smoked) fish.

Supplements which may relieve specific symptoms

Stress, anxiety, mood swings:

Make sure your diet is rich in magnesium, potassium, zinc, essential fatty acids. vitamin C, pantothenic acid. Vitamin B6, vitamin E. Cut out caffeine and sugar. Eat small, frequent meals.

PMS and menstrually-related migraines:

Try evening primrose oil, and make sure you are getting enough magnesium. Vitamin C, zinc. vitamin B6, and niacin (you can buy specially formulated PMS vitamin and mineral supplements from your local health-food store, chemist or supermarket). Take in conjunction with a diet low in animal fat and sugar high in fresh fruit, vegetables and complex carbohydrates.

Menopausal problems:
Make sure you are getting enough zinc calcium.Vitamins A, B, C and E.

Pain:
Make sure you are getting enough magnesium, copper and calcium. Cut down on caffeine. Foods rich in tryptophan (dates, bread, bananas, potatoes, cauliflower) may help, but some migraine sufferers may find these are triggers to attacks.

Nausea:
Vitamin B6 may help.

Herbs
Herbs, although a 'natural' supplement, can be every bit as powerful as prescribed medicines, so they should always be used with respect. Ask for help when you buy from a health-food store: there is often a trained member of staff in the larger stores, who can advise you.They may also be able to refer you to a trained medical herbalist, who can recommend the right herbal remedy for you.

There is, alas, no one great herbal cure-all. Whether or not a herb will give you any relief, it is impossible to say without trying it. For example, I find that peppermint tea is wonderful for nausea and dyspepsia, but unfortunately if it is strong it can trigger a migraine. I find ginger extremely helpful – but that is only my personal experience. My partner, also a migraine sufferer, swears by peppermint and has never had the slightest problem with it. Trial and error is the only answer, I'm afraid! But there is a pretty good chance that your health-food store will yield at least one herbal remedy which can offer you some relief.

Feverfew
Feverfew has long been considered an effective remedy for migraine, and in clinical trials at the City of London Migraine Clinic, 70 per cent of patients said they experienced some improvement in the frequency and/or severity of their migraine attacks.

However, it has now been established that feverfew has its

drawbacks too. Not everyone responds well to it, and in many cases the beneficial effects are accompanied by undesirable side effects, notably month ulcers and inflammation of the mouth and tongue.

The fresh or dried leaves of the feverfew plant (tanacetum parthenium) can be eaten in a sandwich, and many sufferers mix the leaves with lettuce or sprinkle them with sugar, to disguise the bitter taste. The recommended daily dose is one large leaf, or three smaller ones.

Alternatively, you can buy feverfew in tablet or capsule form from a health-food store. This is a more convenient way to take the herb, but it may not be quite as effective. You may need to take feverfew for up to three months before you can be sure whether or not it is helping you.

Feverfew must not be taken if you are pregnant or breast feeding, or by children.

Herbal teas
You can make your own herbal teas by adding dried or fresh herbs to boiling water and letting it stand for five minutes. The recommended amount is two teaspoonsful of fresh herbs per pint of water (or one teaspoonful if using dried herbs). It's advisable to strain the infusion before you drink it, or use a metal 'ball' infuser to hold the herbs.

However, the safest (and least messy) way to use herbs is to buy the commercially produced herbal teas available in bag form from health-food stores. Make sure that you are buying the pure form of the herb, and beware of anything which claims to be a 'blend' or to contain 'natural flavourings'.

The following herbal teas have proved popular with migraine sufferers:

- Lime-flower: if using fresh flowers, make sure they are not wilting.
- Feverfew: avoid in pregnancy.
- Chamomile: relaxing, calming and soothing. May cause nausea if too strong.
- Mint: excellent for nausea, flatulence and other digestive problems.
- Ginger: all forms of ginger are excellent for digestive upsets and nausea. If you can't face ginger root tea, alternatives are

crystallized ginger, or powdered ginger dissolved in warm milk.
- Lavender flower: many sufferers find lavender very calming.
- Rosemary: soothing and relaxing, particularly for ordinary tension headaches.
- Raspberry leaf: quite useful in the days leading up to a period. Ginger and caraway seed teas are useful during menstruation.
- Valerian: helps to ease pain. This is a very strong herb, and it is recommended that you drink only shop-bought teas.
- Hops and catnip: both useful for tension headaches.
- Vervain: useful for tension headaches and migraine. Helps to ease pain.

Exercise, relaxation and lifestyle

It's no good making efforts to eat a healthier diet if you don't also try to modify your lifestyle. What's the point of cooking a healthy, balanced, enjoyable meal if you don't take the time to sit down and enjoy it – slowly? And what's the point of putting the right fuel into your body if the engine doesn't work properly because you never take any exercise?

Exercise
It's no use trying to wriggle out of it with excuses: you and I both know that exercise is good for you, me, all of us. It's perfectly possible to exercise if you are a migraine sufferer, but you must adjust your lifestyle and eating habits to accommodate the new, more active you.

Don't wrinkle your nose in horror! Exercise doesn't have to be a 50-mile hike or an hour on an exercise bicycle, going nowhere. It can be anything from dancing to making love, swimming to a walk in the country. Even if all you do is leave the car at home sometimes and walk to the shops, your body will feel the benefit – and it will thank you for it. Muscles which are regularly and gently exercised will become stronger, more supple and elastic, less liable to go into spasm or to cause a nagging headache which just might turn into a migraine attack.

Preventing hypoglycaemia
It's understandable to be wary of exercise if every time you play

squash, you end up with a pounding migraine. OK, so give up squash – or better, plan ahead so that you don't fall victim to the hypoglycaemia which is probably at the root of the problem. Just before you exercise, take in a little energy. Sugar isn't generally a good idea, but in these circumstances a glucose tablet is ideal – just enough to get you through. When you have finished exercising, make sure that you eat a proper meal as soon as possible. Many migraine attacks are caused by missed or delayed meals: for example, if you always exercise after work and consequently your evening meal gets pushed back two or three hours ... or forgotten altogether.

What sort of exercise?

If you don't usually take much exercise, do consult your doctor before buying the trainers and the leotard. There might be some good medical reason why you shouldn't exercise, but almost everyone can do some sort of exercise, even if it's only a gentle stroll down the road, or one width of the local swimming pool. Your doctor will probably be able to suggest the best sort of low-impact, low-risk, gentle exercise for you.

I have found quite a lot of relief after exercising with small (1.5kg) dumb-bells, to strengthen my arms, shoulders and neck. But again, check with your doctor beforehand; this might not be the right type of exercise for you.

Nowadays there are plenty of beginners' gentle exercise classes for the faint-hearted or the embarrassed. If there isn't one in your area, get together with friends and hire an instructor yourselves!

Learning to relax

Most of us lead lives which are far too hectic, with not enough time to think, let alone pamper ourselves. At the very gentlest end of the exercise scale, you could try yoga, Tai Ch'i, the Alexander Technique or Transcendental Meditation (TM). Or why not attend a relaxation class, or learn self-hypnotism? All these activities will help you to became more aware of your body, and will promote relaxation and suppleness.

It's also a good idea to sit down and think about the way you live your life. Is it more stressful and chaotic than it needs to be? Ask yourself these questions:

- Do I organize my time as well as I could?
- Could my partner help more?
- Do I waste a lot of effort doing things which I don't really need to do?
- Could I cut down on non-essential activities?
- How do I feel about my job? Is it a major source of stress in my life?
- If so, are there any ways in which I could reduce that burden of stress?
- How could I change my life to make it less stressful?
- Am I happy?
- If not, why not?
- Am I unhappy about things I cannot change? Or could I take charge of my future and do something about them?
- Do I have enough time to myself, to think and do the things I want to do?
- If not, can I find time and set it aside?

These are just some of the questions which you could ask yourself. If possible, sit down with your partner and discuss the situation together. Migraine isn't much fun, either for you or your partner. Anything you can do to reduce the number and/or frequency of your migraine attacks will benefit both of you, and your family and friends too; so you have a right to ask for understanding and support. If you possibly can, set aside time for thought, reflection, gentle exercise or simply doing nothing – whatever takes your fancy. Many people – particularly women – feel torn between their own needs and those of their partners, families, colleagues and friends; but we all need time to be ourselves. Make a resolution to take better care of yourself. This will help to improve your self-esteem, and could also help your migraine. And you'll be surprised at how much more other people respect you when you respect yourself!

Take time out to:
- learn relaxation, TM, Alexander Technique or another system to help you unwind;
- pamper yourself: don't feel guilty about those little treats you've been promising yourself for ages. You deserve to have time and

money spent on you!
- set aside time each day, just for yourself. Be firm!
- express your needs;
- take up a new interest;
- organize your time more efficiently;
- plan for attacks, so that you don't feel anxious about the world falling apart if you're ill. That way, the attack may never come;
- if you're not sensitive to strong smells, try aromatherapy. Rosemary and lavender oils can be mixed with massage oils and rubbed in, or dropped on to a handkerchief and inhaled;
- teach your partner massage and/or acupressure.

Chapter Seven

Migraine and slimming

Many migraine sufferers have problems with their weight, and have great difficulty in sticking to a slimming diet because it so often leads to an increase in migraine attacks.

This chapter explains why migraine sufferers find it difficult to diet, and offers some simple, practical advice which may help you to achieve slimming success.

Why do migraine sufferers find it so difficult to diet?

When we begin a slimming diet, this generally means making sudden and dramatic changes in our eating habits.

Frequently, dieting involves exchanging three substantial meals, plus regular snacks, for three much smaller meals and no snacks at all. Often, it also means exchanging favourite or commonly eaten foods for 'healthy' foods we don't normally eat very often.

Some of us, desperate for quick results, may cut out breakfast or lunch; or substitute sugary meal replacements for regular meals. Others resort to frequent cups of tea and coffee, or cans of diet drink to fill up and keep their willpower from flagging.

This common pattern of dieting can lead to all sorts of problems. Take this case study as an example.

Joy's diet

Joy – a lifelong migraine sufferer – was 40, fed up and chronically overweight. She dreamed of shedding her excess pounds, as she suffered from back problems and knew she would feel better if she were a little lighter; but each new diet seemed to end in failure. She had tried dozens of different regimes over the years, but had always given up because it made her feel so ill.

She decided to start her next diet at the weekend, so that she would have time to get used to it without the distractions and temptations she encountered at work; the sandwiches, fizzy drinks, biscuits, chocolates and cakes which her colleagues always seemed to be guzzling all around her.

On Friday night she decided to get rid of all sources of temptation ... by eating them. She ate up all the remaining biscuits and a couple of slices of cake, washed down with a few glasses of her favourite wine.

She slept a little late on Saturday, and decided not to bother with breakfast as she had eaten too much the night before. She felt hungry and a little off-colour during the morning but kept going on black coffee and a couple of cans of diet coke. Lunch was a strawberry 'shake' – a slimmer's liquid meal replacement – as she couldn't face a 'tasteless' meal of meat and salad. She succumbed to a meal replacement bar mid-afternoon, as she had been rushing about and didn't feel too well.

By teatime she didn't feel like eating anything except golden syrup sandwiches: she had a terrible craving for sweet food, and knew that she was building up to a migraine attack.

Where did Joy go wrong?
Joy made just about every mistake in the book

- She started by eating up leftover foods; many of them highly sugared and processed. It's possible some of these may have contained foods to which she was intolerant.
- She overslept, then skipped breakfast. This is not just a bad idea from a blood-sugar point of view; it's also very bad for willpower. Many dieters give up and binge simply because they're so hungry.
- She had a sugary meal replacement for lunch, rather than proper, sustaining food. The high sugar content would have sent her blood sugar level soaring for a short time, after which it would fall dramatically.
- She ate another snack in the mid-afternoon. By now she was probably in the pre-attack phase, and her cravings for sweet foods were a sign of the approaching migraine. They could also indicate withdrawal symptoms.

The migraine attack itself probably resulted from a combination of trigger factors:

- swings in blood sugar levels, caused by fasting then eating too much sugar

- relaxation of stress after a busy week
- disrupted sleeping patterns
- possible withdrawal symptoms caused by cutting out foods to which Joy was intolerant.

The right way to diet

There is no single reducing diet which will suit everyone, but there are certain rules which every slimmer can benefit by following.

Eating the right things

A migraine-friendly slimming diet is one that doesn't involve long periods of fasting. You may well find that you lose weight simply by changing your eating habits and following the healthy eating guidelines suggested in Chapters Four and Six. Because these diets are high in fibre and unrefined carbohydrates, and low in refined sugar and stimulants, they may be easier to stick to as they are sustaining and help to keep blood sugar levels steady.

One of the best ways to stick to your diet is to divide up your calorie allowance for the day into five or six small meals, rather than three big ones. If you space your mini-meals at regular intervals throughout the day, you probably won't feel hungry and you shouldn't suffer from hypoglycaemia.

Most important, always start the day with a decent breakfast. Calories consumed early on in the day are more quickly burned up than calories eaten just before going to bed, so eating a good breakfast won't make you fat and it will set you up for the day. If you miss out on this all-important first meal of the day, by lunchtime you will be hungry, demoralized and may well have the beginnings of a migraine attack.

Avoid eating large meals last thing at night, but do try to have a small, starchy snack before you go to sleep – perhaps a sandwich or a few crackers. This could reduce the danger of waking up with the beginnings of an attack.

Tailoring your diet to meet your needs

One problem with many diet books and diet sheets is that they tend to recommend eating foods that many migraine sufferers prefer to avoid

– for example, hard cheeses and oranges. Clearly, if you're going to cut out cheese, you will need to replace it with alternative sources of protein and calcium; and if you're a vegetarian this can be difficult and a little monotonous. As long as you are not sensitive to dairy products, you can probably avoid cheese problems by sticking to tyramine-free cheeses.

If you are intolerant to a staple food like wheat or milk, you may need to consult your doctor or a nutritionist to draw up an alternative, personalized slimming plan. But as a general rule, most starches have roughly equivalent calorific values, so you can substitute one type of cereal or starch for another without too much trouble.

Getting help and support

It is very important that your diet contains a good balance of fats, proteins, carbohydrates, vitamins, minerals and so on. If you are in any doubt about the nutritional balance of your diet, talk to your doctor: or join a group such as Weight Watchers. Many migraine sufferers have achieved success by joining slimming clubs, which offer tailor-made diets with regular, small meals – and, of course, lots and lots of moral support for the flagging dieter!

Treat private slimming clinics with a healthy degree of suspicion. Some of them do little more than sell you very expensive advice or hand out potentially dangerous slimming pills. Your doctor's surgery may run a weekly weight control clinic, and this is a much safer option, offering both moral support and sound medical advice.

Coping with cravings

If you suddenly stop taking in caffeine, or sugar, or a food to which you have an intolerance, you can expect to experience problems for a short time. These 'withdrawal' symptoms could take the form of cravings, mood-swings or even headaches.

Cut out caffeine slowly, to minimize the risk of rebound headaches. Cravings and other symptoms should disappear when you have been on your diet for a week or so, although some psychological dependence may remain; most of us find chocolate profoundly comforting.

If you are desperate for chocolate, try to work a ration of carob or some other type of confectionery into your diet. Ounce for ounce, toffee is less fattening than chocolate, and it takes a lot longer to eat! But in general, try to avoid eating sugary foods, which will only make your cravings more acute in the long run.

A diet for life

If you suffer from migraine, it is advisable to avoid commercially available slimming products such as Slim-Fast, as these tend to be high in sugar. The sugar may give you a boost, but it won't last long and you may end up with a headache. Even the savoury varieties of diet products are best avoided, as they are frequently packed full of additives.

In any case, the best way to lose weight and keep it off is to make permanent changes to the way you eat. If you accustom yourself to a healthy diet, you are much less likely to backslide once the slimming phase ends: all you need to do to maintain your new weight is eat a little more of what you are already eating.

Pampering yourself

Going on a diet isn't a penance: it's a present from you to your body. You're doing it because you want to feel better about yourself, not to punish yourself for being overweight.

Don't make yourself suffer by making do with boring meals of foods you don't like. Buy specialist cookery books and devise menus that are appetizing as well as quick and simple. The more attractive your food is, the more inclined you will be to eat it – and you'll be less likely to miss the 'forbidden' foods you have chosen to forego.

Exercising

Do take exercise if you can. It will firm you up, and helps to burn up calories. It is also an excellent way of distracting yourself if you feel the need to raid the refrigerator!

However, as a migraine sufferer you need to plan for exercise as sudden strenuous activity may lead to blood sugar problems. Take a small amount of glucose beforehand, and eat one of your small meals soon afterwards. If you plan to do a great deal of exercise, you may need to consider increasing your calorie intake a little.

Dieting success

If you follow all of these rules, it should be possible to achieve a gradual weight loss without exacerbating your migraine. In fact, some people find that their migraines improve a little when they lose weight – although this may be due to improved nutrition rather than simple weight loss. Always remember the migraine dieter's dos and don'ts.

Do

- cut down on caffeine
- give up smoking
- eat lots of fresh fruit and vegetables
- eat little and often
- eat high-fibre, low-fat foods
- eat plenty of unrefined carbohydrates, such as wholegrain cereals
- compensate for any 'trigger' foods which you have decided to eliminate from your diet
- take regular, gentle exercise
- choose a diet which is nutritionally balanced
- take a vitamin and mineral supplement if you feel it is necessary
- avoid constipation
- pamper yourself
- find new activities and interests to take your mind off comfort eating.

Don't

- go for more than three or four hours without eating
- rely on proprietary slimming products, which are often high in sugar and additives
- * drink too many diet fizzy drinks, which may contain caffeine and/or additives such as aspartame and tartrazine
- serve boring foods: make an effort to eat interesting, attractively presented meals to give your willpower a boost
- miss meals
- spend extra time in bed without eating something.

Chapter Eight

Migraine and children

Children can and do suffer from migraine, although parents and doctors may not always recognize it as such.

Since migraine tends to run in families, it's likely that there are other sufferers beside yourself within the circle of your family and relatives; and the chances are that some of these fellow sufferers will be children.

Migraine can be especially upsetting and frustrating for children and teenagers because it isolates them from their peers and prevents them doing all the things they long to do. Just growing up is a big enough challenge, without migraine attacks putting obstacles in your way.

Whether you are a parent, grandparent, aunt or cousin or just a friend to a young migraine sufferer, you can do a great deal, not only to help find the root of the child's problem, but to make the child feel as normal as possible.

Children and migraine

Although most adult migraineurs are female, around 80 per cent of childhood migraine sufferers are boys. It seems that many children grow out of their migraines as they grow up, whilst girls may develop migraine around the time of puberty when their bodies are experiencing large-scale hormonal changes. Stress (for example, exams or parental pressure) may also trigger the first attack in some that are susceptible to the disorder.

Gastric symptoms are especially common in children, with some childhood sufferers experiencing only nausea and vomiting, without the headache. This can lead parents and doctors to assume that the child is just 'nervy' or even making itself sick, although migraine is a common cause and should always he considered.

Doctors generally feel that most childhood sufferers experience common migraine (that is migraine without aura) or abdominal symptoms, although some do suffer from classical migraine (migraine with aura). Some experts, including Dr Howard Freeman, who runs a paediatric migraine clinic at Charing Cross Hospital, disagree with this theory, and believe that children in fact share the same types of migraine as adults, but find it harder to express themselves and describe their symptoms.

Whatever the overall picture, those children who are classical migraine sufferers may find the aura symptoms very frightening and traumatic. Some children may be secretly afraid that they are 'having visions', or going mad.

It is very important for adults close to the child to allay these fears, and to explain that:

- migraine is horrible, but it is not life-threatening no-one ever dies of migraine;
- the pain will only last for a few hours, or a day, and then it will go away completely;
- migraine can be treated, and it will help if the child is a willing partner in that treatment.

If you are a migraine sufferer yourself, you are in a unique position, in that you can talk to the child about your own experiences, your own fears and strategies for coping with attacks. You can also talk about the different ways in which migraine can be treated, and accompany the child on visits to doctors and other specialists.

Is your child a migraine sufferer?

Only a qualified doctor can diagnose migraine, but the following signs may indicate migraine in children:

- regularly complaining of sickness or tummy-ache;
- complaining of difficulty in seeing properly, 'visions' , 'funny patterns','coloured lights';
- tiredness, lack of energy;
- yawning;
- travel sickness;
- bad dreams.

Family links

As we have seen, migraine has strong family links, and in many cases a family will contain several migraine sufferers. Take my own case as an example. My mother and father both suffer from headaches and (in my father's case) abdominal symptoms. My maternal and paternal grandmothers both suffered from migraine, as did my paternal great-grandmother.

All in all, it's perhaps not surprising that I developed migraine as a small child (in fact I can't remember a time when I didn't have it), and – unfortunately for me – it has continued with me into adulthood.

Stress

But are there other possible reasons for developing migraine in childhood as opposed, say, to developing it at puberty or during a time of stress in adulthood? Dr Freeman's views are quite controversial, in that he feels that parents play a role in the development of their children's illness: 'I tend to think that a lot of children would not get migraine unless their parents gave it to them.'

Put differently, Dr Freeman feels that stress is a major precipitating factor in most childhood cases of migraine, and the two main sources of stress in a child's life are school and home. Undue pressure to conform, to overachieve, to be something that the child is not, may lead to suppression of the child's 'forbidden' emotions (anger, fear and so on) and could eventually trigger migraine.

Environmental triggers

We all know that asthma and allergic conditions are on the increase at the moment. Although no-one can be absolutely sure why, it may have something to do with the increase in airborne pollution, or even with the chemical residues in the food that we eat.

These environmental triggers can also have a role to play in childhood migraine; but one of the most important triggers – and one, which it is possible to eliminate completely – is parental smoking.

Many adult migraine sufferers are sensitive to cigarette smoke, and there is some evidence that parents who smoke may have children who are more susceptible not only to respiratory infections and allergies, but to migraine too.

Light

Bright or flickering light can trigger migraine attacks in many sufferers, not just children. I can remember always getting an attack after I'd spent the afternoon fielding in rounders matches and had had to squint into the sun.

But, nowadays, the light trigger is just as likely to take the form of fluorescent lighting, television or computers. Children who are susceptible and who spend a lot of time watching TV or playing computer games may be doing themselves no favours at all.

Food

Doctors acknowledge that food sensitivities can play a part in causing childhood migraine. In trials at Great Ormond Street Children's Hospital in 1982 to 1983, an impressive 93 per cent of the 88 children who took part experienced some improvement in their migraines after following a low-risk elimination-type diet.

However, it's very important not to become obsessive about the diet – migraine link, and this is particularly true in the case of children. Obsessive dieting and the exclusion of foods can lead not only to psychological problems with food in later life, but also to serious nutritional deficiencies. Children need a varied diet, rich in essential nutrients, if they are to grow and develop properly.

Parents may also deceive themselves into thinking that their child's attacks are due to food sensitivities, when the root cause is a more subtle one. As Dr Freeman comments:

Many parents use food allergy to cover up the real reason for the migraine – parental pressures, for example. It's parental escapism... Some parents simply won't recognize it, and don't even come back to a second consultation. They won't accept that it could be due to their relationship with the child.

They go to food allergists and alternative therapists, and spend a lot of money. Of course, migraine is cyclical, and if you go on long enough it will remit naturally... Then the parents will claim that the special diet has worked.

There are certainly practical dangers in overplaying the food angle in children. A child's life – and in some cases, health – can be restricted, deprived and jeopardized by a parental obsession with searching for food allergies or intolerances which simply don't exist.

Low blood sugar

At least as important as food sensitivity – and probably a great deal more important - is hypoglycaemia.

Children lead busy, often hectic lives, with lots of rushing around, bursts of violent exercise, hastily eaten junk food and missed meals. Some refuse point-blank to eat breakfast and display a marked preference for sugary or highly processed foods.

Small wonder, then, that many childhood attacks of migraine are thought to be triggered by low blood sugar levels. Take the example of one individual child.

Lisa's migraine attacks

Lisa (aged 13) was self-conscious about her burgeoning figure and frightened of 'getting fat', even though she was a perfectly normal and healthy shape and size. It was just before her period and she felt 'bloaty' and sore. She decided that she would 'cut down', which meant cutting out breakfast and just starting the day with a couple of cups of strong black coffee.

She set off for school, had a PE lesson and felt ravenous by break. She succumbed to a can of coke and a Mars Bar. She wasn't especially hungry at lunchtime, so she just had a bag of crisps and an orange drink. She ate nothing during the afternoon, as she felt a little sick and was developing a one-sided headache.

It was a stressful day, as she was getting the results of a maths test and was afraid she had done badly. As it turned out, she had passed with flying colours, but by five o'clock, when she finally arrived home after a delayed bus journey, she couldn't have cared less as she had developed a full-blown migraine attack.

Lisa's case shows just how many triggers one child can pack into a single day. Here are some of the factors, which may have precipitated the attack:

- missing breakfast followed by long period without food (low blood sugar)
- strong black coffee (caffeine)

- strenuous exercise on an empty stomach (low blood sugar)
- a can of coke (caffeine, sugar leading to sudden rise in blood sugar levels, followed by possible overproduction of insulin and a dramatic fall in blood sugar level)
- Mars Bar (caffeine, sugar leading to sudden rise in blood sugar levels, followed by possible overproduction of insulin and a dramatic fall in blood sugar level)
- crisps (monosodium glutamate, salt, fat)
- orange drink (possibly tartrazine, sugar)
- long period without nutritious food (low blood sugar level)
- maths test results (stress)
- delayed journey home (stress, low blood sugar).

In addition, Lisa was coming up to her menstrual period, so she was probably at the most vulnerable time in terms of migraine attacks. Obviously this would not be a factor with younger children, but it is easy to see how all those missed meals, sugary snacks, stress and PE lessons could add up to a massive migraine attack.

I have vivid memories of one of my childhood birthday parties – and of a day completely ruined by a migraine attack. The excitement of the party, getting up late and not eating anything so I wouldn't 'spoil my appetite' for the party food, the glare of the July sun, the enormous bar of chocolate . . . all combined to trigger an equally enormous migraine attack.

In many cases, just altering a child's patterns to ensure that healthy, sustaining foods are eaten at regular intervals can make a world of difference to the incidence of attacks. You may not be able to alter your children's hectic lifestyle, but making sure they eat properly and at the right times can make them better able to resist the stresses and excitements which surround them.

Treating childhood migraine

Most doctors are reluctant to put children on long-term drug therapy. The good news is that most children do eventually grow out of their migraine, although some will grow up to become adult sufferers. The most successful treatments seem to combine the following elements

- relaxation
- behavioural modification (reviewing the lifestyle of both parents and child)
- talking to the school to enlist the support of teachers (some of whom may be hostile because they do not understand what migraine entails)
- dietary therapy, not only concentrating on food sensitivities but also on correcting blood sugar problems and ensuring that the child's diet provides all the nutrients essential for good health and normal development.

Protecting your young child

Allergy experts believe that there are certain measures, which you can take, not only to help a child who is already ill, but also to protect unborn children and very young babies from developing allergies as they grow up. These measures may also help to prevent the development of food intolerances and chemical sensitivities – and perhaps also prevent the development of migraine.

Pregnancy and breast-feeding

Breast-feeding provides your child with beneficial antibodies, and may provide some protection against allergies.

However, some experts believe that children can develop food sensitivities even before they are born, if their mothers eat a great deal of a particular food. This could also be the case with breast-feeding, as food molecules (from the mother's diet) are present in the breast milk.

As a general rule, eat a healthy and varied diet during pregnancy, and try to avoid bingeing if you possibly can.

Don't force yourself to eat foods you hate, unless your doctor has told you that they are nutritionally important to you. Don't eat too much of one food, even if you crave it 24 hours a day!

Cutting out tea, coffee, alcohol and non-prescribed drugs will also benefit your child, as will giving up smoking. Eat plenty of protein, unrefined carbohydrates, fresh fruit and vegetables; and take a calcium supplement if you are unable to tolerate cow's milk.

Protecting the older child

Ban smoking from your house, as this will benefit you as well as your child. You may find it helpful to keep the house free from dust and (furry) animals.

Some experts recommend breast-feeding for up to a year. After weaning, make sure that your child eats as varied a diet as possible, and try to keep it additive-free for as long as you can. Try to prevent your child eating too much of a single food. Keep a close watch on sugar intake. Above all, aim for a healthy and nutritious balance of foods.

Never put a child on any sort of diet (elimination or otherwise) without your doctor's approval. If you suspect food sensitivity (e.g. an intolerance to milk), consult your doctor immediately.

Keeping a migraine diary

As with adults, a migraine diary can be a very useful tool to help identify the trigger factors which are provoking migraine attacks.

However, keeping a daily diary is a time-consuming and sometimes tedious process, and it is certainly not something which an unwilling child should be forced to do. It's absolutely vital that you have the complete co-operation of your child, and you will only achieve that if you take time to explain exactly what you are doing, and why. There are very few children who actively enjoy being ill, and most will be quite happy to go along with any scheme if they think there is a chance it will make them well.

Follow the format suggested in Chapter Three when drawing up the diary, but make sure the child is involved in every stage. If they are old enough, there is no reason why children should not compile their own diary, as long as it contains all the necessary information - in a legible form!

Involve your GP too. Once the diary is complete (after a month or two), study it (with your child if old enough) to see if you can identify any likely culprits. Take the diary to your doctor and discuss it with him or her. If necessary, ask for a referral to a migraine clinic and/or a dietician – a good one can help to draw up an interesting eating plan which won't be too restrictive for your child. Any regime which is too repressive, no matter how nutritious, will lead to cheating and bingeing.

Enlist the support of all family members. Ensure that they understand what you are doing, and why, and encourage your child to keep up the good work and not give in. You may find it helps if you and your other children keep diaries too. Set aside regular times each day for filling in the diary, and explain to your child how very important it is that everything goes into the diary . . . including that bar of chocolate they bought with the money they were supposed to spend on fruit!

Elimination diets and children

As a general rule, elimination diets are not a good idea for children, and they should never be used without the support and consent of your doctor. Children have different nutritional requirements from adults, and strict diets could be deficient in vital elements, even dangerous. The golden rules to follow are as follows:

- The moment you first suspect food intolerance, go and see your doctor. Show him/her the evidence in your child's migraine diary, as this may help towards an accurate diagnosis. Make sure the child is examined, to rule out any other causes for the symptoms.
- Ask yourself if there are any other factors, besides food, which may be at the root of your child's migraine. Be honest with yourself. Are there any tensions between you and your child? Do you (consciously or unconsciously) put undue pressure on your child to conform or achieve? Could you be using food intolerance as an excuse to cover up deeper problems?
- Could low blood sugar, rather than food intolerance, be the cause of the problem? If so, try to modify your child's eating patterns so that he or she eats small, frequent meals containing nutritious and sustaining ingredients.
- If you do suspect food allergy or intolerance, don't try to sort out the problem on your own. Never put a child on any sort of diet without your doctor's knowledge and support.
- Never try to put a child on any sort of diet without his/her full and willing co-operation. To do so would be insensitive and could cause the child great distress.
- Use only a diet recommended by your doctor or a qualified

dietician. Don't try to devise one yourself.

- If your doctor recommends an elimination diet, put the whole family on it (and don't cheat!). Show the child that he/she is not alone. This will also help to avoid the problem of other children feeling they are being neglected, in favour of the migraine sufferer. As food intolerance tends to run in families, you may find that several family members benefit from the diet.
- Make sure that family friends also know about the elimination diet, and understand what it is for and how it works. Often, adults think they are being kind to a child by offering chocolate, sweets, fizzy drinks and junk food, but cheating will invalidate the diet completely. Enlist the support of your child, who will probably resist all temptation with a steely resolve as long as he/ she feels involved and really understands what is going on. You may consider offering a reward for sticking to the diet.
- Make sure that your child is getting all the essential nutrients, using a recommended supplement if necessary.
- Remember that there may be distressing withdrawal symptoms for the first few days, and you will have to be strong, explaining why your child must not give in to food cravings.
- If you're not getting anywhere, don't persist with an elimination diet for longer than the period recommended by your doctor. Get skilled help. Food may not be the problem.
- Make sure that your child receives emotional support and does not feel isolated, excluded or deprived. Peer-group pressure to conform can be tremendous, and a child who is made to feel 'different' can suffer secret agonies.

Keeping a sense of proportion

However valuable the dietary approach may be, it is absolutely vital not to lose a sense of proportion. As we've seen earlier in this chapter, parents can sometimes become obsessive, almost fixated on food intolerance as the cause of all their children's problems, even when this patently isn't the case.

The most important thing is for your child to be happy, healthy and emotionally balanced. Feeling cut off from his or her peers will only serve to increase a child's stress levels, and, as we know, stress can be a very powerful migraine trigger.

Even if your child does turn out to have a sensitivity to certain foods, you may find that you don't need to ban them altogether. If your child eats a balanced, trigger-free diet at home, a limited amount of 'banned' food at school, or the odd trip to the pizza restaurant may do little harm.

Don't let restrictions ruin your child's life – keep them to an absolute minimum. The happier, healthier and better integrated your child is, the greater the chance that he or she will grow up to be migraine-free.

Eating to prevent attacks

Prevention is better than cure; and even if your child is not food-sensitive, a good diet may help to rectify hypoglycaemia and any nutritional deficiencies. This can, in turn, help to reduce the incidence and severity of migraine attacks.

Here are the golden rules to follow.

- Make sure your child eats a varied, nutritious diet, with plenty of fruit, vegetables, calcium-rich foods and unrefined carbohydrates for sustained energy.
- Insist that your child eats breakfast and regular meals (or healthy snacks after strenuous exercise) to maintain steady blood sugar levels. This could be a battle of wills at first, but it's important that you persevere.
- As far as possible, avoid processed foods and junk foods. Go for 'safer' fast foods where possible, such as jacket potatoes. But don't become fanatical, and don't exclude all treats: the stress of deprivation may do more harm than that double cheeseburger!
- Try to keep your child off additives, and remember that some medicines (e.g. pain-relieving syrups) contain colourings, artificial flavourings and lots and lots of added sugar.
- Understand the social drawbacks of being a child with migraine, and don't mollycoddle or fuss too much. The pressures can make a child feel alienated from his or her peers and this can cause unwelcome stress. Aim for as normal a routine as humanly

possible. Don't make an issue of things. If your son insists on eating a cheese sandwich and is later ill, maybe next time he'll eat something else! Keeping healthy and avoiding problem foods has to be a voluntary thing, and it's no use nagging.

- Give nutritious packed lunches if school dinners are too much of a minefield. Try to be imaginative if your child really has to avoid certain foods. Use specialist cookery books to create foods your child actually wants to eat. This will require some planning, but many foods can be prepared in batches and frozen for future use.
- Your child is bound to have a migraine attack sometime. When that happens, don't overreact. Be there to offer support, but don't fuss or insist on staying with them if they'd rather be alone.

Try to persuade your child to eat something, however small, in the early stages of an attack, as this may help to abort it or reduce its duration/severity.

FURTHER READING

General books about migraine

Coping Successfully with Migraine, Dyson, S.,Sheldon, 1991, rev. 1993
The Migraine Handbook, Lewis, J.,Vermilion, 1993
Headaches: a comprehensive guide to relief, Lockley, J., Bloomsbury, 1994
The Migraine Revolution, Mansfield, J., Thorsons, 1986
Migraines and Headaches, Petty, R., Unwin, 1986
Migraine (Dr Mike Smith's Postbag), Smith, M.and Kerr. S., Kyle Cathie Limited, 1994
*Migraine Control and Cure,*Walji, H. and Kingston, A,J. R. Reid, 1990
*Overcoming Migraine,*Wyckoff, B., Station Hill Press. New York, 1991

Books about allergy and intolerance

Food Allergy and Intolerance, Brostoff, J and Gamlin, L., Bloomsbury, 1992
*The Allergy Survival Guide,*Houlton, J.,Vermilion, 1993
Allergy: A Practical Guide to Coping, Available by post from Airedale Allergy Centre, High Hall, Steeton, Keighley,WestYorks, BD20 6SB,

Special diet cookbooks and books about healthy eating

No Diet Weight Loss, Walder, P, Wellhouse Publishing 2003
Your Lifestyle Diet Book, Sullivan, K, Wellhouse Publishing 2002
Low Blood Sugar: How to Understand and Overcome Hypoglycaemia, Budd, M. L., Thorsons, 1995
Eat to Beat Low Blood Sugar, Martin Budd and Maggie Budd, Thorsons, 2003
The Foodwatch Alternative Cookbook, Campbell, J.J., Ashgrove, 2003
Not Naughty But Nice, Goddard, L., Ward Lock, 1987
Bumper Bake Book, Greer, R., Bunterbird, 1982

Wheat, Milk and Egg Free Cooking, Greer, R.,T horsons, 1989
Dairy-Free Cookbook, Noble, J.,Vermilion, 1994
Migraine (Special Diet Cookbooks), Norman, C.,Thorsons, 1990
Healthy Eating, Skypala, I.,Wisebuy Publishers, 1988
Diets for Common Ailments, Stanway, P., Gaia, Sidgwick & Jackson, 1989
*The Migraine Guide and Cookbook,*Wentworth, J.A., Corgi, 1982
*Sugar Free,*Wentworth, J.A.,Pawson Books, 1989

Useful Addresses

The Migraine Action Association

(formerly the British Migraine Association)

This is a registered charity with over 14,000 members. They bridge the gap between the migraine sufferer and the medical world by providing information on all aspects of the condition and its management.

The Association has three main aims:

- to provide information and friendly, positive reassurance, understanding and encouragement to migraine sufferers and their families
- to encourage and support research and investigation into migraine, its causes, diagnosis, prevention and treatment
- to gather and pass on information about treatments available for the control and relief of migraine and to facilitate an exchange of information on the subject.

They have a telephone helpline, a quarterly newsletter and numerous leaflets on all aspects of migraine. Members participate in research and product trials and also collect and donate considerable sums of money to support migraine clinics and further research. The Association is funded entirely by donations and members' subscriptions.

Contact details:
Unit 6
Oakley Hay Lodge Business Park
Great Folds Road, Great Oakley
Northants NN18 9AS

Tel: 01536 461333
Fax: 01536 461444
E-mail: info@migraine.org.uk
Website: www.migraine.org.uk

Action Against Allergy

Action Against Allergy was established in 1978 to help those suffering from any kind of allergy. It's aim is to advance understanding, awareness and recognition of allergic medical conditions and allergy-related illness, and the actions needed for research, diagnosis and treatment.

The charity has contact details of allergy clinics, allergy specialists and dietitians, (both NHS and private) and alternative heath-care practitioners. There is a comprehensive list of books on allergies, special diets, treatments and a library of information leaflets. This information service is available for a small donation. You can join AAA for an annual subscription.

Contact details::
PO Box 278
Twickenham
Middx. TW1 4QQ

Tel: 020 8892 2711
E-mail: AAA@actionagainstallergy.co.uk
Website: www.actionagainstallergy.co.uk

Airedale Allergy Centre

Airedale Allergy Centre is a leading treatment centre for those suffering from allergies, intolerances and chemical sensitivities. with a team of dedicated and highly experienced staff.

Contact details:
41 Devonshire Street
Keighley
West Yorkshire BD21 2BH

Tel / Fax: 01535 603966
E-mail mail@airedale-allergy.co.uk
Website: www.airedale-allergy.co.uk

The British Institute for Allergy and Environmental Therapy

(formerly The Institute of Allergy Therapists)

The British Institute was formed to bring together a group of Therapists who were practicing a unique system of allergy diagnosis and treatment. It's members are qualified health professionals both mainstream and complementary. The diagnostic method is simple and without discomfort, the treatment method is by way of homeopathic desensitization and are suitable for infants and children as well as adults.

Contact details:
Ffynnonwen
Llangwyryfon, Aberystwyth
Ceredigion SY23 4EY

Tel: 01974 241376
Fax: 01974 241795
E-mail: mailto:allergy@onetel.net.uk

Transcendental Meditation

24 Linhope Street
London
NW1 6HT

Tel: 08705-143733 between 10am –5pm Monday –Friday
Website: www.transcendental-meditation.org.uk

Yoga

The British Wheel of Yoga
25 Jermyn Street, Sleaford
Lincs. NG34 7RU

Tel: 01529 306 851
Fax: 01529 303 233
Email:information@bwy.org.uk
Website: www.bwy.org.uk

Index

additives 25, 50, 86
allergy therapists 64
analgesic headaches 15
applied kinesiology 38
aura 11-13, 101, 102
– without headache 13
auriculo-cardiac reflex 39

basic elimination diet 55, 57

challenging 48
chemical sensitivity 30, 62
children 17, 101-110
Chinese Restaurant Syndrome 16
cluster headaches 13, 20
combination headaches 13
coping with attacks 102
cravings 67, 68, 96, 98, 99, 110
cytotoxic 36, 37

desensitization 64-66, 117
diaries 109
dietary supplements 82, 87
dining out 68
dowsing 38
drinking 73

elemental diets 59
elimination diets 109
– children 109
environmental control units 64
enviornmental triggers 25, 61, 103
enzyme potentiated desensitisation 66
exercise 74
expert help 63

fast food 46, 54, 71
fasting.. 19, 25
food 19, 25
  – addiction 29
  – allergy 25
  – children.. 104
  – cravings.. 62, 68
  – dining out... 68-69
  – food families 60, 75
  – hidden intolerance 29
  – intolerance............... 6, 27-31, 35-39, 47-53, 66
  – sensitivity 26
  – substitutes.......................... 55-57, 63, 73-75
  – triggers 10, 24, 35, 47

hair analysis 38, 39
hangovers 16
healthy eating 53
herbal remedies 87
hypoglycaemia 85
  – children.. 105
  – exercise 74

ice cream headache................................ 16

medicines.. 51
migraine: attacks 10, 13, 14
  – in children.. 101
  – diagnosis....................................... 116, 117
  – diary 40-47, 52, 54, 108, 109
  – in the elderly 18, 60, 87
  – environmental factors 11, 21
  – heredity... 18
  – illness............... 21, 32, 82, 87, 103, 116
  – in men 12, 18
  – neurological theory 10
  – posture... 15, 21, 83
  – sleep disturbance........... 11, 19-21, 25, 30, 40-44, 97
  – smoking 20, 52, 100, 103, 107, 108

– stress 10, 11, 15, 17, 20, 43, 44, 101, 103
– symptoms 9-14
– triggers 10, 18, 35-40, 47-66
– vascular theory 9
– with aura 12, 102
– without aura 11, 101
– in women 18, 20, 84, 85, 87, 93

pregnancy and breastfeeding 107
prick and patch testing 35
processed meats headache 16
provocation and neutralization 65, 66

RAST test 36
relaxation 92, 93
restaurants 69, 79

scientific trials 27
shopping 72
slimming 20, 22, 42, 95, 97-100
specialists 10, 14, 63, 102, 119
sublingual provocation and neutralization 66
substitute foods 74-80

tension headaches 14-15, 91
– diet 15
testing 35, 36, 38, 40, 47, 48, 54, 55, 58
threshold dose 30
triggers 10, 18, 19, 21, 24, 35, 47, 61, 103

vasco-active foods 49
vega testing 38

Other titles available from

Wellhouse Publishing

HOW TO COPE SUCCESSFULLY WITH

ANXIETY AND DEPRESSION

Beth MacEoin

We live in stressful times and have to cope on a daily basis with a variety of different pressures. These can include financial worries, emotional stresses, bereavement, break-up of relationships and insecurity at work. When feeling well and resilient we are able to cope with a wide range of these stressful situations. It is when we become mentally and emotionally overloaded at a vulnerable time in our lives that we can suffer from symptoms of anxiety or depression. Beth MacEoin describes in her easily accessible style the various symptoms and suggests a wide range of practical measures to provide positive support.

ISBN: 1-903784-03-4

128pp

HOW TO COPE SUCCESSFULLY WITH

CANDIDA THE DRUG-FREE WAY

Jo Dunbar

Candida is the common name for an overgrowth of yeast organism known as *Candida Albicans*. Candida appears with many seemingly unrelated symptoms – it affects almost every part of the body and has become an umbrella term for any collection of symptoms of no identified cause. Because of the wide range of symptoms and the lack of positive diagnostic tests available, this gap has provided fertile ground for individuals of limited medical training to quickly hop on the band wagon and begin 'diagnosing' Candida for almost any condition or illness. This book introduces a thorough drug-free treatment program, as well as tips on how to adapt your life-style to treating Candida.

ISBN: 1-903784-11-5   128pp

HOW TO COPE SUCCESSFULLY WITH

COLITIS

Dr Tom Smith

We know a lot about the changes that occur in the bowel of people with colitis and how to return them to normal. It should be only a matter of time before we know *why* these changes happen. Colitis means 'inflammation of the large bowel' (the colon), inflammation takes several forms and doctors have different views from the general public on what constitutes colitis. Most of this book is devoted to ulcerative colitis and Crohn's, with chapters on how to distinguish these inflammatory bowel diseases from irritable bowel, diverticular disease and colon cancer.

ISBN: 1-903784-12-3   128pp

HOW TO COPE SUCCESSFULLY WITH

CROHN'S DISEASE

Dr Tom Smith

Although on Crohn's disease, this book compares the similarities and differences to ulcerative colitis. Dr Smith describes how modern medicine is used to relieve and prevent serious complications. He explains how the normal bowel works, how it can go wrong and why it can produce the three main symptoms of diarrhoea, bleeding and mucus. This book describes the tests, investigations, and the diagnosis of the illness. It is not just the illness but how much of the bowel is infected that affects the treatment and how quickly and completely recovery is made. Other bowel problems that mimic Crohn's are described.

ISBN: 1 903784 16 6

112pp

HOW TO COPE SUCCESSFULLY WITH

DEPRESSION

Dr Tom Smith

In his easily accessible style Dr Tom Smith describes depression and explains why we get depressed, the treatment with drugs together with other treatments. It shows how to think through your depression, what you can do for yourself and how to change those negative thoughts, become more outward going and assertive together with sleep problems. Depression is a serious illness that needs serious attention. Everyone in the family doctor's team has to help, the sufferer's family must also be aware of the risks and how to give assistance. Dr Tom Smith describes in this book the help you can get.

ISBN: 1903784 14 X

112pp

HIGH BLOOD PRESSURE

Dr Duncan Dymond

Blood Pressure is not a disease, everyone has a pressure, we need it to keep us upright and alive. Your blood pressure varies depending on your level of physical and mental stress. In this easily accessible book Dr Dymond describes what high blood pressure is, the symptoms, various medications available, side effects and possible complications. The tests and investigations for high blood pressure are explained together with treatments and suggestions for changes to lifestyle and diet.

ISBN: 1-903784-07-7   128pp

HIGH CHOLESTEROL

Dr Tom Smith

We are all becoming more aware of high cholesterol problems and often only discover that we are at risk when having a geneneral health check. In this book Dr Tom Smith describes in his easily accessible style the causes of high cholesterol, the associated problems, the complications and the risks involved if your high cholesterol goes untreated. Dr Tom Smith details the treatments available together with possible side effects. He also gives information on diet and lifestyle changes which may be needed to help reduce your cholesterol levels and reduce the risks to your overall health.

ISBN: 1-903784-09-3   128pp

HOW TO COPE SUCCESSFULLY WITH

IRRITABLE BOWEL SYNDROME

Richard Emerson

Irritable Bowel Syndrome is a complex problem with both physical and psychological symptoms. The aim of this book is to set out clearly and concisely these symptoms and the various treatments now available – conventional, complementary and alternative. Ths should enable sufferers to improve their lifestyle and either cure or manage their Irritable Bowel Syndrome.

ISBN: 1-903784-06-9   128pp

HOW TO COPE SUCCESSFULLY WITH

MENOPAUSE

Dr Joan McClelland

The menopause is an event to welcome, a stimulating new chapter in your life. You can say goodbye to period pains, water retention, PMS together with a host of psychological problems including irritability, depression and chronic tension. The menopause is a vantage point from which to take stock, reviewing your earlier life and looking ahead to new interests, deepening relationships and fresh goals. You are entering an important and fascinating time in your life and to get the best out of it you need to work in harmony with nature, this book aims to help you achieve this aim.

ISBN: 1-903784-05-0   128pp

HOW TO COPE SUCCESSFULLY WITH

PANIC ATTACKS

Karen Sullivan

Panic attacks are a much more common problem than is generally realised an affect a large proportion of the population. They can manifest themselves in many ways including agoraphobia, anticipatory anxiety, separation anxiety, school or work phobia. This book explains what Panic Attacks are, the causes, how panic affects daily life and the associated disorders. Conventional treatments together with their side effects are explained and alternative remedies including acupuncture, homoeopathy, reflexology, massage are covered. Karen Sullivan gives reassuring short term measures to help deal with an attack and, together with other advice, Top Ten Tips to help cope in the longer term.

ISBN: 1-903784-08-5   128pp

HOW TO COPE SUCCESSFULLY WITH

SLEEPING WELL – THE DRUG FREE WAY

Beth MacEoin

Good sleep is an important part of your total health. There is no uniform pattern to sleep problems, a great deal depends on an individual's make-up. Problems include difficulties in switching off, frequent waking and a sense of being unrefreshed on waking. Other factors may be over-reliance on caffeine, alcohol or chemical sedatives. Bad working habits can play a large part in preventing sound sleep. This book contains positive strategies to solve these problems and break the negative cycle. The major systems of alternative medicine included in this book have a different perspective to conventional medicine on the issue of sleep problems.

ISBN: 1 903784 13 1   128pp

HOW TO COPE SUCCESSFULLY WITH

STRESS

Anna Rushton

Stress is about change and how we deal with it when we live in a society where there are many changes happening in rapid succession. In this accessible book AnnA Rushton describes Stress. explains the chemical changes that happen to your body and shows how to identify signs of Stress including a Stress assessment chart. AnnA describes what professional help is available and explains what self-help options there are including: Diet & Nutrition, Exercise, Lifestyle Changes, Stress Management, Relaxation Time, Alternative Therapy guide plus Top Tips to handle your Stress.

ISBN: 1 903784-18-2   128pp

HOW TO COPE SUCCESSFULLY WITH

STRESS AT WORK

Beth MacEoin

In the UK we work longer and harder than our counterparts in Europe and America. Working under pressure has an adverse affect on our health and manifests itself in many cases as stress. It is now accepted that a reasonable amount of stress is a good thing and essential to motivate us and to trigger the 'fight or flight' response we sometimes need to deal with exceptional situations. Excessive stress can be extremely harmful and may in some cases cause death, for example the over pressurised Sales Rep speeding to their next appointment. This book contains positive strategies to solve these problems to break the negative cycle and enable you to re-assess your overall work situation.

ISBN: 1 903784-15-8   128pp

THYROID PROBLEMS

Dr Tom Smith

The thyroid is not a subject that immediately springs to mind when we chat socially about our health. We marvel how some people have boundless energy while others are always tired and weary. There are nervous, anxious, agitated people who can never sit still. It is easy to assume that people differ in these ways because of their characters or lifestyle but a substantial number have developed these characteristics through no fault of their own. These are the sufferers from thyroid problems. Do Tom Smith describes in his easily accessible style the symptoms, different types of thyroid problems, complications and the various treatments available today.

ISBN: 1-903784-01-8   128pp

YOUR LIFESTYLE DIET

Karen Sullivan

A healthy diet is more than just balancing food intake, it involves eating foods that promote rather than endanger health. What are the elements of a healthy balanced diet? How do we identify which are good fats, bad fats and essential fats? What problems can be caused by sugar in our diet? What are the different types of sugars found in our diet and which are healthy? What should we drink and what should we avoid drinking? What essential supplements do we need? The answers to these questions and many more are contained in Your Lifestyle Diet.

ISBN: 1-903784-04-2   128pp